ADVANCE PRAISE

"*Reimagining Healthcare* is a must-read book that focuses on the most significant global health influencers: women. Through her important research, Carolyn Buck Luce—a strong advocate for empowering women to make the best possible health decisions for themselves and their families—has established that women are the linchpin for health and wellness. We were excited to be part of this important research with our colleagues from the healthcare industry. It showed that the healthcare industry must change the way it engages and communicates with women to provide them with the knowledge and confidence they need. This is an especially important lesson for health communications agencies and their partners. Communication is the cure, and women are listening."

—Lynn O'Connor Vos, CEO, ghg | greyhealth group

"For too long, our healthcare systems and providers have fallen into viewing their missions through the wrong end of the telescope, focusing on 'sick care' over healthcare and narrow specialties rather than whole human beings. In *Reimagining Healthcare: Through a Gender Lens*, Carolyn Buck Luce advances a realistic set of solutions, centered on the hidden, universal strength of global healthcare—the roles of the women who serve as strategists and decision-makers at every level, from patient, through family, to leadership in key healthcare segments. Carolyn's insights are framed by her long and illustrious experience as a brilliant business analyst and, just as importantly, through her remarkable journey as a caregiver. This is a compelling read from one of healthcare's most highly passionate—and compassionate—thinkers."

—Freda Lewis-Hall, MD, DFAPA,
Executive Vice President and Chief Medical Officer, Pfizer Inc.

"Now more than ever, the healthcare industry is in need of novel solutions to address inadequate care and rising costs. *Reimagining Healthcare* offers a comprehensive, fact-based, and global argument that the solution is already there...women. It's a compelling and overdue wake-up call for healthcare leaders to embrace and fills the missing puzzle piece for next generation customer-centricity."

—Brian Goff, former President of Hematology, Baxalta

"*Reimagining Healthcare* makes a convincing case that healthcare companies need a new approach to women, their biggest market and their biggest employee group. With hard data and clear examples, Carolyn Buck Luce (healthcare and human resources expert, mentor, and colleague) describes how the industry must think and act differently to improve health outcomes. Her book will challenge your current beliefs and also help you to think differently about your role in transforming healthcare."

—Kimberly Park, Worldwide VP,
Customer Strategy and Innovation, Merck

REIMAGINING

THROUGH A GENDER LENS

HEALTHCARE

REIMAGINING

THROUGH A GENDER LENS

HEALTHCARE

CAROLYN BUCK LUCE
FOREWORD BY SYLVIA ANN HEWLETT

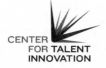

CENTER
FOR TALENT
INNOVATION

This is a Center for Talent Innovation Publication

A Vireo Book | Rare Bird Books
453 South Spring Street, Suite 302
Los Angeles, CA 90013
rarebirdbooks.com

Set in Minion
Printed in the United States

10 9 8 7 6 5 4 3 2 1

Publisher's Cataloging-in-Publication data

Names: Buck Luce, Carolyn, author | Hewlett, Sylvia Ann, 1946-, writer of
foreword.
Title: Reimagining healthcare : through a gender lens / Carolyn Buck Luce ;
foreword by Sylvia Ann Hewlett.
Series: Center for Talent Innovation
Description: Includes bibliographical references and index. | First Trade
Paperback Original Edition | A Center for Talent Innovation Publication | A
Vireo Book | New York, NY ; Los Angeles, CA: Rare Bird Books, 2016.
Identifiers: ISBN 978-1-945572-25-8
Subjects: LCSH Health care reform—United States. | Women's health
services—United States. | Women's health services—Marketing. | Medical
care—Sex differences. | Health—Sex differences. | Social medicine. | Medical
policy. | Discrimination in medical care. | Medicine—Research—Sex
differences. | Delivery of Health Care. | BISAC SOCIAL SCIENCE / Research
| SOCIAL SCIENCE / Disease & Health Issues | MEDICAL / Health Care
Delivery | MEDICAL / Health Policy
Classification: LCC RA564.85 .L83 2016 | DDC 362.1082—dc23

To the courageous change agents who have been at the
heart of this research:

Kimberly Chappell
Laurie Cooke
Lynnette Cooke
Grace Figueredo
Lisa Gutierrez
Wanda Hope
Laurie Kowalevsky
Kimberly Park
Katherine Johnsen Read
Eiry Wyn Roberts
Meredith Ryan-Reid
Aida Sabo
Catherine Sohn
Lynn O'Connor Vos
Donna Wilson

PROJECT TEAM

Project Leads

Carolyn Buck Luce, Executive in Residence

Sylvia Ann Hewlett, Founder and CEO

Writing and Editing

Melinda Marshall, EVP, Director of Publications

Dan Horch, Fellow

Quantitative Research

Laura Sherbin, CFO, Director of Research

Pooja Jain-Link, Senior Research Associate

Charlene Thrope, Research Associate

Qualitative Research and Production

Julia Taylor Kennedy, SVP, Director of Digital Learning

Isis Fabian, Research Associate

Catherine Chapman, Research Associate

Communications

Tai Wingfield, SVP, Director of Communications

Silvia Marte, Senior Communications Associate

CONTENTS

FOREWORD

Whats getting in the way of good outcomes when it comes to patient health?

Not simply rising costs, nor elusive cures.

Rather, what may be keeping people from regaining or maintaining their health is the industry's failure to enlist and engage its most crucial customers: women.

The industry does so at its peril. The most significant emerging market in the world is not China, but women. As consumers, but also as highly qualified employees, women are powerful determinants of competitive strength—a fact affirmed by two of our recent studies conducted by the Center for Talent Innovation. In 2014, with *Harnessing the Power of the Purse,* we explored the clout of the female investor in China, Hong Kong, India, Singapore, the UK, and the US; in 2015, with *Power of the Purse: Engaging Women Decision Makers for Healthy Outcomes,* we investigated women's impact on health in Brazil, Germany, Japan, the UK, and the US.

Carolyn Buck Luce, who led the 2015 study and coauthored the resulting report, knows a thing or two about healthcare and the role women play in delivering it. To our endeavor she brought decades of experience, both as EY's global healthcare sector leader and as her family's Chief Medical Officer. She knew, from first-hand experience, that when it comes to health, women call the shots. They set health and wellness agendas for themselves and for their families, choose treatment regimens, and see that everyone takes their meds or keeps doing their physical therapy exercises. Women are the ones hiring and firing doctors, pharmacists, and insurance providers. So it was pretty clear to her that the industry had better earn their trust—and after we surveyed more than nine thousand people in Brazil, Germany, Japan, the US, and the UK, it was clear the industry had failed to do so.

In this book, derived from our report, Carolyn lays out a plan for industry leaders to forge that connection. With our data and powerful stories from the field, she makes the business case for "gender smarts"—how empowering women on the inside of the industry can help it better connect with women on the outside. And with examples of initiatives at major pharmaceutical companies, she shows leaders what gender smarts look like: how companies might engage women as consumers and harness their insights as healthcare professionals. Promoting women into industry leadership roles, she argues, will accelerate the industry's transition from product-centered to patient-centered models.

Carolyn's solution for healthcare industry leaders simply underscores the message that she and I have been sharing with multinational leaders in the Task Force for Talent Innovation for the last twelve years: market growth depends on not just workforce diversity, but also on diversity in leadership. Tapping women for their insights, and greenlighting women's ideas on how to reach and serve female consumers, demands that companies have inclusive leaders—leaders who listen to the quietest voice in the room and give traction to ideas they may not personally relate to. Inclusive leaders, we find, are likely to be people who embrace difference, whose experience has conditioned them to perceive the power of difference. Companies with diverse leaders, our research shows, are more effective in capturing and keeping growth markets. Gender-smart leaders are the ones poised to capture the world's biggest emerging market (3.5 billion women and growing).

Industry leaders who heed Carolyn's call to action will enjoy a first-mover advantage. But there's enormous benefit to the rest of us if we empower and support women as decision makers, innovators, and leaders: we're likely to be healthier. With women in charge of our health, we're going to eat right, take our vitamins, exercise regularly, see the right doctor when we're ill, finish the medicines we're prescribed, and heed the protocols proven to help get us better.

That's an outcome we should all be willing to fight for.

—Sylvia Ann Hewlett, Founder, CEO,
Center for Talent Innovation
September 2016

INTRODUCTION

The healthcare industry has a solution, at its fingertips, to some of its most intractable problems—but it still hasn't grasped that solution.

Its most dominant market segment consists of customers and end users who share needs that cut across health condition, age, ethnicity, nationality, education, and income—but the industry isn't focused on this segment.

The needs of this dominant segment are understood and shared by many employees inside healthcare companies, including at senior levels. But their insights into their own demographic are rarely solicited.

Who are these insightful employees? Who are these customers? And what is the solution for the industry's future growth?

Women.

Women comprise 59 percent of patients and make 80 percent of all decisions affecting patients in the US.[1] Women make up 88 percent of healthcare professionals and, as mothers and wives and daughters, 66 percent of caregivers.[2] Women are also the super-consumers: they control $29 trillion in worldwide spending—expected to increase to $40 trillion by 2018[3]—and account for 80 percent of healthcare purchases in general and 93 percent of OTC pharmaceutical purchases.[4] In fact, the "SHEconomy" is the dominant force driving the industry to abandon its current model—which centers on disease, specific product offers, and opaque pricing—and adopt a "patient-centric" model that is responsive to individual patient preferences, needs, and values.

Healthcare executives do recognize the cost savings and health benefits of a patient-centric model. In 2011, a CapGemini report predicted patient centricity would help pharmaceutical companies increase adherence rates.[5] In 2012, EY's *Progressions* report, which I co-authored, said the movement would disrupt healthcare business models globally by prompting new approaches to product research and development, nudging patient behavior, and forging collaborations with other industry players.[6] McKinsey predicted that patient centricity would prompt hospitals to try to modify patient behavior,[7] alter pharmaceutical companies' relationships with doctors and other medical professionals,[8] and spur the electronic availability of data and personalized medical information.[9] A.T. Kearney cited a few early-stage efforts by Pfizer and Johnson & Johnson and called for pharmaceutical companies to adopt a health-outcomes focus in their offerings.[10]

Certainly the executives I've spoken to recognize that the disease- and product-centered model is broken. The evidence, after all, is incontrovertible:

- *Approximately 50 percent of prescribed medicines are not taken by the patient.*[11] *Even after pharmaceutical companies have succeeded in proving a medicine's worth to doctors, and even after doctors have communicated that value to patients and written them a prescription, the sale and the cure aren't taking place.*

- *Two thirds of new pharmaceutical products fail to meet pre-launch sales expectations.*[12] *Even after new treatments have passed lengthy and costly scientific and regulatory hurdles, they fail in meeting expectations far more often than they succeed.* Much of the industry's $135 billion in annual research and development spending[13] isn't optimized—even when the treatments are scientific successes.

- *Penalties under the Affordable Care Act for high hospital readmission rates in the US are rising, not falling.*[14] *Despite some exemplary exceptions, hospitals as a whole aren't moving fast enough to keep patients healthy and avoid the need for expensive, repetitive care.*

But executives are nonetheless slow to adopt this model. With the exception of some insurers and pharmaceutical companies, the industry remains stolidly within its business-to-business (B2B) comfort zone. The sheer size of the global healthcare market—$8 trillion, and still growing faster than inflation[15]—makes transformation a daunting project. Add to this scale an ever-tightening web of regulations and delivery constraints, and it's easy to see why the pace of change is glacial.

Yet healthcare consumers, empowered by technology and unprecedented access to information, are growing impatient. Armed with app-rich smartphones, and accustomed to instant gratification of their every need through Google and Amazon, consumers expect and demand better healthcare options. They see no benefit to being loyal customers. As better choices become available, they're inclined to switch to them.

Hence to survive, let alone prosper, the healthcare companies of today must not only adopt a patient-centered model, but also understand—and meet—the needs of their most important customer segment.

Women.

NOT JUST CUSTOMERS, BUT CMOs

To help companies get a clearer picture of this vital segment, I led a research study for the Center for Talent Innovation (CTI), where I am executive in residence. The study moved us from "anecdata" to globally relevant findings and affirmed that women's importance to the industry goes far beyond their value as super-consumers.

To better understand women as consumers, the industry needed, we posited, a new kind of market analysis. Our path forward was informed by author Clay Christensen's famous idea: people buy products or solutions because they need them for a specific job, not because they themselves belong to a traditional socioeconomic demographic.[16] In healthcare, people's "jobs" are: taking care of their own health; caring for others in illness; and making healthcare decisions for others.

In the resulting report, *The Power of the Purse: Engaging Women Decision Makers for Healthy Outcomes*, we demonstrated that women perform not just the first two jobs, as everyone knows, but the third, too: they make healthcare decisions, not just for themselves, but also for spouses and partners, children, parents and in-laws, and other family members and loved ones.

These women are, in effect, Chief Medical Officers (CMOs). They choose which medicines to buy and which treatment regimens to follow. They also act as Chief Nutritionist, Chief Physical Trainer, Chief Pharmacist, and Chief Veterinary Officer. They are the ones who make sure that everybody, including the patients and caregivers, does their job. As CMOs, they have the power to fire those who underperform—doctors, hospitals, pharmacists, and insurers.

I would know, because I'm one of them.

My late husband was diagnosed with esophageal cancer in 2006. The doctors gave him three months to live, but neither of us was willing to accept that. As generally happened with healthcare questions in our family (as in most families, all over the world), I became the decision-maker: the CMO. "I'm the battlefield, and you're the general," my husband told me.

As CMO, I researched clinical trials for experimental treatments for my husband, and I got him into them. To choose the best hospital, I interviewed doctors and surgeons. When it became necessary, I made the call to switch doctors and hospitals. I engaged with the insurance companies in what felt like a contact sport, and when I couldn't get what I wanted, I switched insurers mid-stream. I went to all of my husband's appointments and made many of the decisions necessary both to prolong his life and retain the quality of his life during chemotherapy, which is so painful and difficult for both patient and caregiver. And I did this while working a full-time, demanding job and guiding our four children through this difficult passage for our family.

At the end, my husband let me make the decision about when to call a stop to treatment, so that I could deliver on my promise that he could die among his loved ones, at home. We'd managed to give him three good years of life and love.

I was lucky. At the time of his illness, I was a principal and global leader of the Life Sciences sector at EY, responsible for a $1 billion professional-services business serving pharmaceutical, biotech, and medical-device companies around the world. My years in the healthcare industry gave me knowledge and contacts that few people have. Even so, during this ordeal, the last place where I could find help and guidance in making a good decision was a pharmaceutical or insurance company. They provided neither useful websites nor knowledgeable and caring employees I could talk to. I found that many of our doctors were unprepared, unable, or unwilling to guide me in my decisions. The best source of information turned out to be my informal network: the women healthcare leaders that I had met through the Healthcare Businesswomen's Association (HBA) and my client work. They gave me their "unofficial" guidance, along with their empathy and support.

I share this story because, as the research I conducted at CTI makes abundantly clear, women aren't asking the industry for new medicines, which are often costly to generate. Rather, as CMOs, they are asking for a new relationship. They want providers who are committed to and engaged in the shared mission of improving health outcomes—not just pushing more products. They want companies to understand the many roles they perform and arm them with what they need in order to do their CMO jobs well. And they want partners who can solve for the three famines from which nearly all of them are suffering: time, trust, and knowledge.

As you'll see in forthcoming chapters, women do not have these things.

THE DISCONNECT

Why is that?

With women making up the majority of healthcare professionals,[17] you'd think the industry would be more in touch with their needs and wants. But interviews I've conducted with senior women in healthcare businesses point to two stubborn problems: women aren't well represented in leadership, and those who do make it to the top wish to be seen as executives, not as caregivers.

I'm Exhibit A. For all that my husband's illness taught me, for all that I learned about the system's failures, and for all the ideas I had that might correct for those failures, I never shared any of these ideas with clients or colleagues. In fact, only when I convened members of the HBA for a focus group did I learn that my ordeal as a CMO was not only common, but that, like me, none of these powerful women had ever shared their takeaways and insights with other leaders at their companies.

The reason? Because as one senior executive explained—a woman whose company produced Alzheimer treatments and yet who felt like she was "winging it" as caregiver to her Alzheimer-afflicted mother—women who've managed to climb to the top tiers of management in healthcare want to be seen as wholly committed professionals. "I'm afraid that I might be seen as unable to manage that professional role if people know what I also have to manage at home," this CMO explained to me.

"We're all CMOs, but we don't show up as CMOs at work," Kimberly Chappell, director of Multichannel Management for US Medical at Bristol-Myers Squibb, told me. "We have insights, but we aren't sharing them. There's concern about how much sharing is acceptable."

"Women try to fit into the corporate image of what a leader is," Laurie Cooke, CEO of the Healthcare Businesswomen's Association, shared with me. "Since the majority of role models are men, women often choose to leave their female, nurturing side behind for the sake of their workplace brands. I've seen many women avoid showing a sensitive side as they try to project that they're as tough as the man sitting next to them. What a loss to the organization to miss out on a more nurturing culture with authentic leaders."

Kate O'Connor, executive director of communications at Boehringer Ingelheim, cited legal concerns when I brought up this phenomenon with her. "Companies may not want employees sharing too much about personal healthcare matters," she said. Still, the cultural element resonated with her, too. "At work, I want to be known for running a business, not running a household," she said. Then she added, "But it is also an important responsibility of women in leadership roles to foster an environment where women can bring their whole, authentic selves to work, particularly as the lines between work and life are increasingly blurred."

INSIDE AND OUTSIDE, WOMEN ARE THE SOLUTION

The problem that these women articulate points to a ready-made solution, both for consumers and healthcare providers.

If companies get smart about inviting and using the knowledge, insights, and experiences of their women employees, they might find ways to adopt a customer-centric model that wins over women as patients and CMOs—improving outcomes, boosting revenues, and gaining a competitive advantage in the global marketplace.

Catherine Sohn's story illustrates how. When she was director of vaccine products for US Pharmaceuticals at SmithKline Beecham (now GlaxoSmithKline), she learned that aid workers in many developing countries were giving multiple vaccine doses all at once, since local conditions often made it impossible for patients to return at precise intervals. It was immediately clear to her that a combination vaccine, one that delivered several therapies with a single application, would be a great boon for the developing world.

And it was also clear to her, when her global vaccine committee debated whether there was a market for a combination vaccine in the developed world, that she had the answer as a result of being the CMO for her family.

"I realized, it was a pain for me to go in multiple times to get my kids vaccinated," she says. "If we could increase convenience while maintaining efficacy, as the R&D department had demonstrated that we could, then the potential wasn't just in developing countries. It was here in the US, too, for mothers of small children."

Sohn shared her insight, and the committee voted to develop the combination vaccine. Its success prompted GSK to develop and sell combination vaccines all over the world.

Her story goes to show that when companies train leaders to adopt the inclusive behaviors that elicit and endorse women's insights and ideas, the results can be significant. In fact, CTI research shows that when senior leaders at publicly traded companies both embody diversity (are inherently diverse) and have learned to embrace difference in others (have "acquired diversity")—what we call two-dimensional (2D) diversity—employees are 45 percent more likely than employees at companies lacking diversity to report that their companies have grown market share in the last year. They're also 70 percent more likely to report that their companies captured new markets in the past year.[18]

"Women play a leading role as 'chief medical officer' for themselves and their families," says Wanda Bryant Hope, chief diversity officer at Johnson & Johnson. "Engaging women in the workforce helps drive innovation and connection with this critical decision maker."

The vast majority (78 percent) of employees that we studied in our 2013 study, however, say that leadership at their companies lacks both inherent and acquired diversity,[19] and thus their firms are not reaping these returns.

THE NEXT GREAT OPPORTUNITY

The next great market for health companies starts with the women inside their ranks.

Smart companies will not only continue to hire, train, and promote women; they'll create an inclusive culture that makes it easier for these women to share their insights as CMOs. In this inclusive culture, more women will assume leadership roles; with women in leadership, more women coming up the ranks will feel empowered to share their insights to drive innovation for the industry's dominant market segment. As the connection is restored between C-suite executives and family CMOs, the industry can at last deliver on its promise of improving the health of billions, one person at a time, by winning over its most important customer group for the long term at a relatively low cost.

Empowering women on both the inside, as leaders, and on the outside, as CMOs, has the potential to fulfill what patient-centric healthcare has long promised:

- increased *adherence* to prescribed regimens, which boosts *return on innovation*;

- decreased costs associated with managing acute and chronic diseases, *bending the cost curve*;

- a *quicker* "time to patient";

- *brand enhancement* through increased customer insight and engagement;

- greater *engagement and retention* of female talent as women feel valued, heard, and invested in;

- a richer pipeline of *insights*, where more ideas from women win the endorsement needed to become *market innovation*; and

- *improved outcomes*, which burnish *corporate reputations*.

A company that wins on both the inside and the outside will be poised, as well, to capitalize on the next generation of talent and consumer: Gen Y and Gen Z. These future consumers of healthcare will demand that the industry be dramatically different. They want healthcare, not sick care.[20]

For all of these reasons, industry leaders need to get "gender-smart": to understand women as not merely patients with specific diseases but also CMOs; as not merely caregivers but also employees with valuable insights to share. In this book, drawing on robust data, focus group insights, interviews with industry leaders, and countless conversations with women, I offer them guidelines.

There's no time to lose. The stakes for the industry and the opportunity for the health of society have never been greater. Today, we have a vicious cycle:

- CMOs have to make decisions without the tools they need, leading to...

- distrust of an industry that brims with life-saving knowledge and committed people...

- who rein in their ambition as their passion and knowledge go untapped.

A change in approach can unlock these frustrated energies, beginning a virtuous cycle that will reinvent the healthcare industry.

PART ONE:
HEALTHCARE TODAY

1

Know Your Consumer

During my years at Ernst and Young, one thing became crystal clear to me: when companies incorporate a patient-centric model, health outcomes and corporate bottom lines improve.

The difficulty is that this model requires more than a statement of intent or a top-down directive. It requires that healthcare companies understand how a patient and her family live with a condition—the tensions and frustrations they experience, the perspectives they bring. It requires mapping how a condition impacts patients' lives as a whole. It requires looking at a typical patient's emotional state at key stages and inflection points of her life's trajectory. It also requires looking at who is influencing and/or making the actual decisions about treatments, activities, schedules, options, and alternatives.

Eli Lilly and Company's launch of Forteo, a treatment for osteoporosis, in Japan, shows how this model can work. "It was the fastest and most successful launch of Forteo anywhere in the world," says Eiry Wyn

Roberts, vice president of Chorus and Exploratory Medicine at Lilly.

Lilly's success with Forteo is especially noteworthy since, prior to launch, several aspects of the drug indicated that it might be a tough sell.

To work as it is supposed to and reduce a patient's risk of fracture, Forteo requires daily injections. But administering daily shots is intimidating for most patients. And convincing patients to take these shots during the months or years when they don't have any symptoms—osteoporosis rarely presents symptoms between fractures—was likely to be a very difficult task. After all, people often can't be bothered just to take pills as preventative care.

But clinical trials showed that the drug was highly effective. So Lilly adopted a new marketing approach.

The company decided to target not just the Japanese women diagnosed with osteoporosis. The firm targeted their daughters and daughters-in-law as well. Lilly's marketing team understood that women usually make healthcare decisions for the whole family and, more often than not, adult daughters take responsibility for managing their mothers' health.

So Lilly accompanied Forteo's launch in Japan with an online campaign called "Itamiru" ("See Your Mother's Pain"), which included a website—still live today—with medical, nutritional, and treatment information for caregivers of osteoporosis patients. The site encourages daughters to learn more about the causes of back pain, identify the signs and symptoms of osteoporosis, locate a specialist nearby, fill out a health assessment form with their mothers, and bring it to an Itamiru-branded clinic or hospital.

Since 2012, the site has received 270,000 visitors, and Lilly estimates it has helped to bring the medicine to approximately 4,000 extra patients who need treatment to reduce the risk of dangerous bone fractures.

"It's an approach that's led not only to better, more enduring relationships for Lilly with consumers and those who care for them," says Roberts, "but most importantly provides an enhanced opportunity for improved outcomes for patients. It has helped us understand the patient—her thinking, her needs, and her decision-making process—in a very different way, so we can position our product to speak to those needs."

WOMEN CALL THE SHOTS

Lilly in this case did what a wealth of market research urges: they got to know their consumer. The healthcare industry has known for years that women make the majority of decisions in healthcare. But the research I led at CTI shows that, to succeed with women, it's vital to understand how culture and lifestyle factor into their decision-making. Companies also need to know the types of decisions women are making, for whom they're making them, and what influences their decisions.

In every market, women are in charge of their own disease management. As patients (and 74 percent of the women in our survey reported having had an illness within the past year), 94 percent make healthcare decisions for themselves.

What the CTI research makes clear, however, is that women are making decisions for loved ones as well as for themselves: 94 percent of working moms* make decisions for others; so do 33 percent of single women who don't have children. Often these decision makers are also caregivers, looking after adults currently suffering from illnesses, or for children who have long-term illnesses. Just over a fifth (23 percent of stay-at-home moms and 22 percent of working moms) say they're caring for children with long-term illnesses; 31 percent of stay-at-home moms and 47 percent of working moms report they're caring for adult relatives.

When women make decisions for others, they're doing far more than just overseeing or administering care for the treatment of a disease. Women are also safeguarding health and well-being, setting the agenda for themselves and their families with regard to nutrition, fitness, screenings, prescriptions, supplements, and taking many other actions that add up to wellness. That encompassing approach to healthcare is one that women are keen that the industry understand—and facilitate.

---

* Defined in our survey as employed women with any children under the age of 18. Stay-at-home moms in our survey are defined as women who are not employed and who have any children under the age of 18.

Figure 1.1
DECISION MAKERS VS. CAREGIVERS
(All markets)

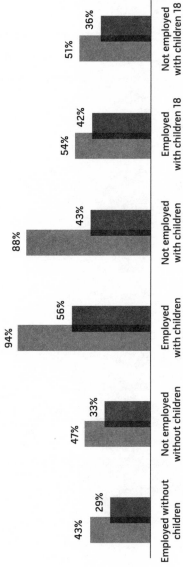

Employed without children — 43% / 29%

Not employed without children — 47% / 33%

Employed with children under 18 — 94% / 56%

Not employed with children under 18 — 88% / 43%

Employed with children 18 or older — 54% / 42%

Not employed with children 18 or older — 51% / 36%

Women who make health and wellness decisions for others
Women who are caregivers for others

2

How Women Define Health

Women have a holistic definition of health: more than avoiding sickness, health for women is about physical fitness and emotional and spiritual well-being.

The industry professes interest in this vision, but has yet to embrace it fully. If they did, I'm absolutely certain that they would find many opportunities to improve health outcomes and customer loyalty.

Risa Lavizzo-Mourey is an example. Lavizzo-Mourey grew up eager to help others thrive. She watched her father, a physician, treat young and old African American patients in their Seattle community. She watched her mother, the medical director of a neighborhood health center, work to make sure that lower-income patients had access to healthcare. "All of those things came together to give me an interest not only in practicing medicine but in keeping people healthy," Lavizzo-Mourey says.

After graduating medical school, she entered geriatrics and found it rewarding: "Families will never forget it if you get it right with their aging parents,"

Lavizzo-Mourey says. But in working with the elderly, she grew increasingly aware of how the system limited the care she could give—and she also grew frustrated with how the system privileged and neglected certain groups, how it worked, and how it created obstacles to healthier lives. "To really make a difference, you realize that focusing on the patient right in front of you, as satisfying as that is, isn't enough," she says. "You can often do more if you start thinking about how you can change the system to enable that person to get what they need. You keep moving upstream as it goes, and that was my career trajectory."

So Lavizzo-Mourey decided to enter the field of public health—and her career took off. She eventually became president and CEO of the Robert Wood Johnson Foundation, the largest philanthropy focused on health in the US, with support from the likes of First Lady Michelle Obama and PepsiCo CEO Indra Nooyi. Through RWJF and the communities it supports, Lavizzo-Mourey is working to create what she calls Cultures of Health.

"That means having high-quality, easy-access healthcare," she explains. "But it also means building a community that encourages healthy choices in the way you live your life, from where you work to the schools your kids go to. It means that people who make policies make it easier for you to become fit, to walk, to bike, to have transportation that gets you to and from a job that allows you to have a healthy lifestyle and make enough money to have a living wage. Cultures of Health encompass all those things that enable us to be healthy, including those things that help us be connected spiritually and emotionally."

Lavizzo-Mourey's holistic vision of health encompasses, our research shows, how most women in our five-country sample define health.

SICK CARE ISN'T HEALTHCARE

The Oxford English Dictionary defines health as "the state of being free from illness or injury." The Merriam-Webster Dictionary similarly focuses on health as "the condition of being well or free from disease."

Likewise, pharmaceutical companies and health systems tend to define health as the absence of illness. It's evident in their structures: divisions focus on discrete diseases or disease categories. Physicians specialize in a single part of the body or family of diseases. But the women interviewed said that health for them means far more than treating illness.

"I don't think about curing, but caring," a registered nurse from São Paulo, Brazil, said. "I am focused on my mother's quality of life," a caregiver in Osaka, Japan, explained. "Health is all about lifestyle and living actively," a working mom in Los Angeles reflected.

Female physicians, too, saw their roles in more holistic terms. "For my patients, what's happening in their lives may be more important than what's happening to their bodies when it comes to what they think about 'health,'" a rheumatologist said. Other physicians similarly insisted that women patients could not be treated as an assemblage of parts. "You have to see her as a whole person, and treat her from a whole-person standpoint," an OB/GYN explained. "When care of a woman starts getting fragmented, it takes a long time to diagnose things—because things are missed."

Figure 2.1
WOMEN DEFINE HEALTH AS...
(All markets)

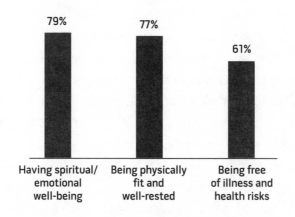

79%	77%	61%
Having spiritual/ emotional well-being	Being physically fit and well-rested	Being free of illness and health risks

In our study, nearly everyone agreed: health means having spiritual and emotional well-being, and being physically fit and well-rested. When given a list of options, time and again, respondents gravitated toward these definitions. In all markets surveyed, 61 percent of women include being free of illness in their definition of health. Yet 79 percent include emotional and spiritual well-being, and 77 percent include physical fitness.

Digging into the data, while the percentages vary slightly, the rankings are fairly consistent: across country, class, ethnicity, gender, and generation, respondents overwhelmingly include physical fitness and emotional and spiritual well-being in their definitions of health—far more often than they include being free of illness.

Curing or preventing illness, it would appear, isn't sufficient for health. Women want to be well, physically, mentally, and emotionally. "Women do think more about health than illness, and look for ways to promote health instead of fix illness," says Jo Taylor, chief customer officer and vice president of Global Market Research at Eli Lilly. "As an industry, I believe we have a unique opportunity to understand and address the implications of this."

HOW THE INDUSTRY DEFINES HEALTH

Many of the women we interviewed for this study shared stories that underscore how women's definition of health departs from the industry norm. Alexa Meara's story stands out in particular. A rheumatologist, Meara treats illnesses like lupus and rheumatoid arthritis, chronic diseases that disproportionately affect women. Treating these diseases is particularly challenging, she finds, because they are associated with crippling fatigue that can interfere with every aspect of women's lives. The medications are commonly associated with significant side effects, too.

One of Meara's patients at Ohio State University, a woman who suffers from scleroderma, recently confided in Meara that she just can't see socializing with her friends anymore because of her dry mouth and swallowing difficulties. "She was in tears in my office," Meara relates. "She says, 'I can't go out to dinner with friends because I'm afraid to eat, and then I look like I don't eat. So I just don't go out anymore.' Those are the kinds of outcomes my patients are focused on: whether they can live normal lives."

At Ohio State University, Meara says she is one physician among many intent on providing healthcare that not only addresses symptoms, but that also restores quality of life. Yet the healthcare industry, she says, is currently unable to study quality of life as a primary outcome—instead, companies must demonstrate improvement in how a patient feels, functions, or survives.

Fatigue, for example, is very important to patients but difficult to connect to measurable outcomes. Meara explains that it's critical to understand all of the measureable components of fatigue, not just how tired a patient may be, or how much sleep is gained or lost. "For example, lupus patients, ninety percent of whom are women, are always concerned about fatigue, yet doctors rarely include it as an outcome measure," Meara says. "Fatigue is a complex symptom that we need to learn more about in order to develop the correct outcome measures for it. We don't know how to fix it. I can check on how many hours you've slept, but helping your tiredness doesn't necessarily help you deal with ongoing fatigue."

Others share Meara's concern that the treatment perspective in healthcare is too narrow, with its focus on treating discrete symptoms. "Most of my patients are healthy in the traditional sense of the word," says Monica Svets, an OB/GYN at the Cleveland Clinic. "What they really need is help managing stress, anxiety, depression. I can provide an ear for them, and occasionally help with a prescription here and there, but they're looking for the system to provide more support for those mental health and wellness solutions."

Amy Compton-Phillips, chief quality officer at The Permanente Federation, the umbrella organization linking eighteen thousand physicians practicing with Kaiser Permanente, agrees. She says that patients want a "medical home," a place that will treat them for more than a single health concern. To that end, she's working to ensure that Kaiser Permanente moves away from the "doctor-per-body part" model. "We have, I believe, as a society, become so overly medicalized that we have a hard time meeting people's holistic health needs," she reflects. "Because we want to test and treat every little discomfort, we have gotten away from how to stay healthy and balanced through all stages of life."

SUCCEEDING WITH A HOLISTIC APPROACH

When Tokyo-based pharmaceutical company Eisai Co. Ltd. prepared to launch its breast cancer drug, Halavan, in the US, it decided to take a holistic approach.[21] Breast cancer and its treatment infringe significantly on women's day-to-day well-being and their ability to care for family members and others. So the company explored ways not just to deliver the drug to patients, but to supplement it to address their broader lifestyle challenges.

The company discovered that the number one concern for breast cancer patients is their limited ability to pull together a nutritious dinner for themselves and their families, given the nausea and fatigue that accompany cancer treatments. Clearly, "health" for these women means prioritizing not just an effective course of treatment for themselves, but also figuring out how to meet their CMO responsibilities. So, in 2012, Eisai decided to start a meal delivery program specifically for breast cancer patients: Magnolia Meals at Home.

Participants receive ten meals per month that, in keeping with a holistic approach to health, are uniquely designed to help satisfy the nutritional needs of breast cancer patients. If requested, they can receive an additional ten meals for family members, all delivered directly to their homes. The meals are frozen and contain a label with a meal description, expiration date, ingredients, nutritional information, and cooking instructions.

Eisai has partnered with key community and advocacy organizations which identify eligible patients, obtain their consent, and refer them to the program. Then, the Meals on Wheels Association of America takes over, reaching out to participants to set up a schedule and deliver meals directly to their homes. Eisai employees also volunteer to help distribute meals and, in certain instances, deliveries include assistance in carrying and storing food. In working toward alleviating concerns about providing food for family members, Magnolia Meals at Home aids in patients' health and well-being outside the realm of sick care.

Currently, Magnolia Meals at Home has helped more than one thousand families in New York, New Hampshire, New Jersey, Massachusetts, and North Carolina. It's been so successful that last year it was expanded to include thyroid cancer patients too. "I enjoy preparing my meals, but some days I'm too tired, and Magnolia Meals at Home comes to the rescue," said one patient.

This concern for wellness, as opposed to just symptom treatment, is beginning to spread. Meara applauds work done by Outcome Measures in Rheumatology (OMERACT), an independent consortium of international health professionals that is trying to change the way outcomes for medicines are measured so that the measures better reflect patient priorities. The Federal Drug Administration in the US is already taking into account OMERACT's more patient-friendly outcome measures when evaluating rheumatology drugs for FDA approval.

Hospitals, too, can do more to put patients at the center of care. Maureen,* whose son suffers from a rare

---

* Indicates name change to ensure source's anonymity, here and throughout the rest of the text

brain condition, interviewed two children's hospitals to decide where to send him for a risky surgery. Boston Children's Hospital sent her to a series of appointments with specialists at the tops of their fields to consider the different elements of his care. Yale–New Haven Children's Hospital, in contrast, set up a single meeting with a group of specialists around a table with Maureen and her son to construct a collaborative approach to his care. "It was a no-brainer, I went with Yale-New Haven. I felt so much more comfortable that they were putting his needs first and working as a team to produce the best outcomes," Maureen says.

Eisai, OMERACT, and the Yale-New Haven approach are steps toward a more holistic consideration of health. Were this holistic mindset applied throughout the industry, our research suggests, it would align healthcare professionals with healthcare consumers in ways that benefit both. As chronic conditions are the leading cause of death around the world, it becomes vital that every interaction—from conversations about treatment in the examination room, to outcome measures from the FDA for clinical trials, to marketing at a pharmaceutical company—take into account women's point of view: that healthcare must maintain or restore quality of life, and not simply address the symptoms of disease.[22]

And to understand women's point of view, it's crucial to understand women in their decision-making roles as Chief Medical Officers.

3

The Chief Medical Officer:
A New Lens on the Market

Lynnette Cooke is chief executive officer of consulting and market research company Kantar Health, but her responsibility as a health executive doesn't end there. She also makes certain her young son and husband stay current in their health assessments, eat nutritious meals, exercise regularly, and, when they fall ill, get the best medical care. She does the same for herself. Increasingly, she's overseeing care for her elderly mother as well as for her sister, who has a severe developmental disability and lives in a group home with peers.

She is, in short, Chief Medical Officer of her family, with responsibility for half a dozen people whom she loves.

It's a big job. Helping to manage the health of her mother and sister is particularly tricky, as Cooke is in New York, while her mother is in Florida and her sister is in Michigan. Constantly on the telephone with her mother's and sister's doctors to get updates, Cooke is often frustrated by the doctors' reluctance to really talk with her about the different possible treatment options. "If I question a regimen, my mother's doctor sometimes takes the attitude of, 'Well, what would you like me to prescribe for her?'" she explains. "I almost feel that I am put in the position of the educated expert, instead of the other way around."

In her sister's case, Cooke fears that the number of specialists her sister sees are not coordinated in her treatment. Because her sister is unable to articulate her symptoms, it's hard for her doctors to diagnose the root causes of health issues that crop up. Cooke regularly uses vacation time to visit her sister and mother, and to check in with their doctors and local health support services. That leaves precious little time to manage the healthcare and wellness of her own family, especially as Cooke often travels for work.

To make time for her son, she blocks time on her calendar as she would for any other chief-executive activity, isolating the 4:30 p.m. to 7:00 p.m. slot to be home while he is doing his homework and to make dinner for her family. "I do a lot of nine p.m. calls and early morning starts to make this work," she says. "But I am fortunate that I get to set my schedule without feeling guilty. And no one will give me a hard time because I get my work done." She adds, "Unfortunately, this kind of flexibility is not as easy for a lot of women trying to look after their family's well-being."

I certainly empathize with Lynnette. Beyond the difficult journey of my late husband's last chapter of his life, I'm the mother of four children. When they were growing up, I was constantly on call as the CMO. One of my sons suffered from a tumor in his hip that required five operations and three rounds in a body cast. Another was born with Kleinfelter's syndrome, a rare chromosomal condition that causes a range of learning disabilities and physical symptoms, made worse by the early onset of Type 1 diabetes. A third son skied off a cliff during my late husband's illness and broke his back. I'm also the CMO for my eighty-eight-year-old mother.

Today my children are all adults in their thirties, and they still call me with questions that I nearly always have to answer on my own, because there's no "go-to" place that I can turn to for help. Every call obliges me, as CMO, to do original research and act as a health and medical detective at the same time that I'm working long hours at my career.

And just as I am for my family, the women we interviewed act as advocates, proxies, and decision makers for their loved ones, as do a majority of the women (59 percent) we surveyed—in short, they qualify as Chief Medical Officers. These women, 71 percent of whom are married or living with a partner, not only determine their own healthcare: as CMOs, they ensure that family members and other loved ones are taking their medications, eating well, and creating healthy lives. They make the decisions about compensating, hiring, and firing doctors, pharmacists, insurance companies, and pharmaceutical companies.

Figure 3.1
THE CMO...
- DECIDES FOR PATIENTS
- DELEGATES TO CAREGIVERS
- HIRES AND FIRES HEALTHCARE PROFESSIONALS

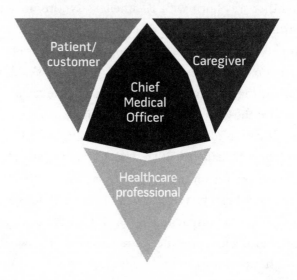

CMOs are, in short, healthcare companies' most important consumers. If the CMO is engaged, respected, and included, she'll speed the industry's transition to a patient-centered, well-care-focused business model. Yet in board rooms, in examining rooms, and in policy discussions about healthcare, the mother/daughter/sister/friend who shapes others' health outlook and daily health habits is rarely acknowledged, supported, or respected as a crucial decision maker and patient influencer, let alone understood as a consumer.

FROM LIFE STAGE TO LIFESTYLE: THE KEY TO THE FEMALE MARKET

A few vanguard companies are beginning to think about the CMO. Typically, they perform a life stage assessment of her responsibilities and preferences, creating what's referred to as a "patient journey." Merck, for example, launched a qualitative research effort in 2012 with women of multiple generations to better understand the family's "Chief Wellness Officer." Merck's marketing team sought to study women as they move through life's different stages: when they might live independently, when they might get married and have kids, when they might start worrying about eldercare for their parents, and when they might retire and confront more health issues of their own. By identifying the resources these wellness officers need to make the decisions they're called upon to make, Merck has taken an important step toward engaging the CMO and harnessing the power of her purse.

These "life stage" analyses are a step in the right direction, but women's decisions about marriage, childbearing, work, and retirement no longer conform to predictable decades of their lives. Our research shows that dividing CMOs according to their life circumstances or lifestyles gives a far better picture of their decision-making habits and unmet needs.

Industry professionals agree: life stage is not necessarily indicative of life circumstance. Dawn Halkuff, vice president of marketing and sales in Women's Health at Pfizer, knows from personal experience—she's a single woman without children—that her preferences and attitudes can't be discerned by looking at her age and stage. She sees a competitive advantage for Pfizer in favoring lifestyle assessment over life stage analysis. "It's a fascinating shift in industry thinking," Halkuff says. "And it's the next opportunity for us in terms of better understanding those women, thereby communicating much better with them and serving them better."

Our survey shows that life stage analysis fails to account for huge swaths of the female market. If the industry were to assume, for example, that women in their 30s will be married with kids, it would miss the 61 percent of thirty-something-aged women who aren't married or don't have kids. If the industry were to assume that caregiving doesn't begin to hit women until their forties, it would miss 37 percent of the women who are providing care or acting as decision makers for adult relatives—women who are under forty.

Figure 3.2
WOMEN WHO ARE CMOs†

	% who are CMOs
Employed women without children	43%
Not employed women without children	47%
Employed women with children under 18	94%
Not employed women with children under 18	88%
Employed women with children 18 or older	54%
Not employed women with children 18 or older	51%

† Working = Employed full time, employed part time, and/or self employed. Stay-at-home/ not employed = Not employed and not looking for work, retired, long-term disability, and/or homemaker. Children under 18 = Women with at least one child under the age of 18. Children 18 or older = Women with children who are all age 18 or older

Understanding the CMO depends on understanding the life situation she navigates. When women in the survey were divided into six key segments, the results showed that throughout all segments, large numbers are serving as CMOs (see Figure 3.2). Some results may be particularly surprising. Yes, working mothers are likely to be CMOs making decisions or caring for kids and adults. But working women without kids are also likely to be looking after the health of others.

Working moms have a different set of constraints and concerns than stay-at-home moms do. Despite their double shifts, working moms often take on broader decision-making responsibilities on behalf of their loved ones. Take vaccinations: 75 percent of working-mom CMOs make vaccination decisions on behalf of others, versus 66 percent of stay-at-home-mom CMOs. When it comes to scheduling, 72 percent of working-mom CMOs make scheduling decisions for others, in comparison to 66 percent of stay-at-home-mom CMOs.

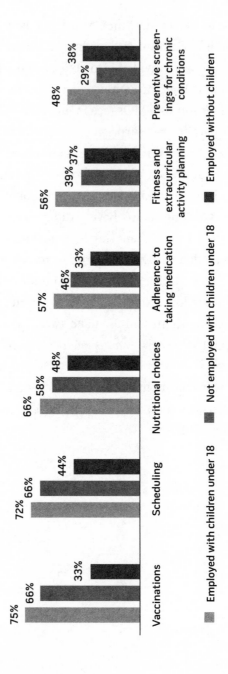

Figure 3.3
WHAT TYPES OF WELLNESS AND ILLNESS DECISIONS HAVE YOU MADE FOR OTHERS?
(Female CMOs, all markets)

While it may seem counterintuitive, this finding didn't surprise the working moms. "If you need somebody to get something done, you ask a busy person," says one CEO of a nonprofit and mother of five. Think of Lynnette Cooke—the efficiency she has honed through years of juggling responsibilities and making quick decisions as a workplace leader is the same efficiency she applies to her CMO responsibilities at home.

Meanwhile, a substantial number of working women CMOs without kids are also calling the shots: 33 percent make vaccination decisions for others—including spouses, partners, parents, in-laws, and other family members and loved ones—and 44 percent make others' scheduling decisions.

Other interesting insights about these decision makers emerge from an analysis of the data by country and by ethnicity. For example, significantly more Japanese and Brazilian women make decisions for others than do women in the US, UK, and Germany.

Figure 3.4
WOMEN WHO MAKE HEALTH AND WELLNESS DECISIONS FOR OTHERS

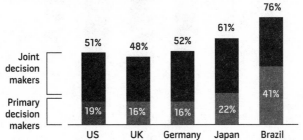

"Women are usually the ones with the final say in Japanese households," affirms Keiko Sheriff, leader of market research at Eli Lilly in Japan (see page 49 for more on the Japanese CMO).

In the US, more Asian and Hispanic women are making decisions for others than white or black women are. This difference has significance for how patients and their families can best be approached. "I encounter people—some who work at healthcare companies—who still think men rule the Latino family," says Venus Ginés, founder of Dia de la Mujer Latina, a large US network for patients of breast cancer. Ginés is also a passionate health activist on behalf of Latinas. "They don't understand that Latina women are in charge of health. I don't think the industry has captured that yet, and that's a shame."

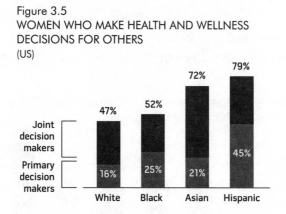

Figure 3.5
WOMEN WHO MAKE HEALTH AND WELLNESS
DECISIONS FOR OTHERS
(US)

Household income level also leads to certain nuances. With the exception of women in Brazil, women in the top household income bracket are more likely to make decisions on behalf of others than those in the lowest household income bracket because, as one focus group participant observed, "access to means simply brings more purchasing power." This phenomenon is, once again, most pronounced in Japan (where 61 percent of women are decision makers for others).

THE CONFIDENCE DEFICIT

Despite such nuances, CMOs have, as consumers, quite a lot in common. Healthcare companies might view them, in fact, as universal customers. For example, no matter who these women are, and no matter what their family circumstances, most feel overwhelmed and ill-equipped to do the job of making health decisions for their families.

Across all markets, 58 percent of CMOs aren't confident that they're making good health and wellness decisions for their loved ones. This lack of confidence is even pronounced in developed markets: 64 percent of CMOs in Germany don't think they're making good decisions; neither do 91 percent of CMOs in Japan. Confidence does vary according to lifestyle circumstance—45 percent of working moms aren't confident in their health decision making, as compared to 66 percent of stay-at-home women without children—but this self-doubt is common enough to be a defining trait.

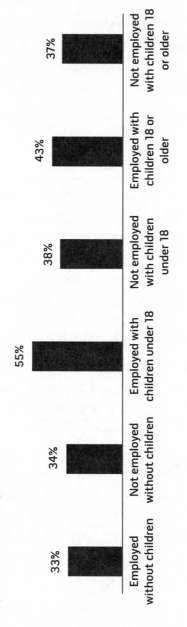

Figure 3.6
WOMEN WHO ARE VERY CONFIDENT THEY MAKE GOOD
HEALTH AND WELLNESS DECISIONS FOR OTHERS
(CMOs, all markets)

What causes this self-doubt are the three famines of time, knowledge, and trusted industry partners. The ways in which these deficiencies create obstacles for women, depending on their lifestyles, will also point the way toward their solutions.

4

Three CMOs' Stories

KEIKO SHERIFF, CMO IN JAPAN

In some ways, women who identify as CMOs in Japan (as 61 percent do) have an easier job of it, thanks to the nation's comprehensive healthcare system. "My son's school arranges for regular checkups, which include vision and hearing tests, for his general health maintenance," explains Keiko Sheriff, leader of market research at Eli Lilly in Japan. "Plus, my husband and I get regular checkups from our workplaces. The system makes us do health maintenance, so as a mom, I just have to make sure I get regular reports."

But in other ways, because of societal expectations of women (50 percent stay home, as compared to 35 percent in the other countries we studied), Japanese CMOs have it harder. "Since men are traditionally the breadwinners, women in Japan are expected to take care of everything at home—probably more so than in other cultures—from prevention and healthy living to finance to caregiving when a family member is sick," Sheriff explains.

Overseeing nutrition and providing healthy meals is a big part of the job. Sheriff recalls preparing a bento box for her son to take to school when he was young and she was living and working in the US. Though she worried he would be teased for bringing it, she was more worried there wouldn't be a nutritious alternative (and in fact, his lunch got eaten by the other kids; Sheriff recalls him asking her to make two so that he could share).

Now that her son is back in school in Japan, she trusts that his school meals are nutritious, so that's one responsibility off her plate. But her concern about his nutrition has prompted her to hire someone to cook three healthy meals at a time, which Sheriff can warm up for dinner so she can manage her work and life balance better. "This kind of outsourcing is still not commonly utilized in Japan, but as more women begin to work outside of the home, it is becoming slightly more common," she says.

For healthcare companies, the Japanese market presents several contradictions. On the one hand, the integration of healthcare into work and school brings major convenience to working women; on the other, they incur social penalties for outsourcing responsibilities around nutrition and prevention.

The convenience of the nation's system makes it easy to obtain prescriptions to treat family maladies; but that ease coupled with the affordability of prescription medication can cause a high volume of visits to the doctor. "In Japan, we go to the doctor for any little thing," Sheriff observes. "Not only do people want to be seen by doctors right away for some reason but also because it's far cheaper to get a prescription from the doctor than to buy an over-the-counter medication, and the prescription will be stronger."

As healthcare consumers, Japanese women, too, present contradictions. For all the responsibility they bear for the health and wellness of their families, very few express confidence in their abilities to do the CMO job well. Only 9 percent of them think they are making good health and wellness decisions for their loved ones, compared to 50 percent of CMOs in the other four markets we studied. Japanese women also report the lowest levels of trust in healthcare professionals in our survey, and are least likely to profess knowledge about healthcare.

Sheriff, who in her marketing role frequently polls Japanese respondents, isn't surprised by these findings. "Japanese people simply won't choose five on a five-point scale," she explains. "Culturally, we have a tendency to avoid 'extremes' and also consider a four excellent. It's a generally observed tendency in Japan."

URSULA VON DER LEYEN, CMO IN GERMANY

Working mothers have long had an uneasy role in German society. It's only in the last ten years that many German schools have extended their days into the afternoon. In our sample, only 23 percent of German

CMOs are working women with children under eighteen (on the low end of the markets we surveyed). Still, the number is on the rise. As more and more mothers work in Germany—41 percent of German mothers with young children now work, according to the OECD—they look for role models that can show them how to navigate work and family.[23]

Politician and Federal Defense Minister Ursula von der Leyen serves as one. Mother of seven, and with a father suffering from Alzheimer's disease, her ability to succeed as a high-powered career woman and take care of her family's health and well-being makes others aware of new possibilities for the German CMO. "I know I am a good mother," she tells *The New York Times*.[24]

By outsourcing some childcare to nannies and cleaning to housekeepers, von der Leyen sets an example for middle-class mothers who can't afford to stay home and raise their children full time. Her conservative politics shield her from accusations of radical feminism, and despite garnering her share of critics, she also has become something of a media darling; newspapers have called her "Supermom" and "Mother of the Nation."[25]

One key to becoming "Mother of the Nation" has been sharing her experiences. In an interview with *Die Welt*, von der Leyen admitted the difficulties she faced in caring for her father as his symptoms of Alzheimer's progressed. But while she delegates certain tasks in her role as CMO, she strives to prioritize familial relationships. "When I think about how much my father helped me along life's path, I find it natural to help him at the end of his life," she tells *Die Welt*.[26]

In her openness as a public figure juggling profession and family, von der Leyen demonstrates how a fulfilling career doesn't diminish her ability to also serve as CMO—it simply changes her approach to the role.

AMANDA HINCHCLIFFE, CMO IN THE UNITED KINGDOM

Each morning, Amanda Hinchcliffe makes sure her children, her husband, and an uncle with Down syndrome have what they need for a productive, healthy day—while also getting herself out the door for a full-time job. When her uncle suffered a stroke that brought on permanent dementia, it became an overwhelming burden to balance his needs with those of the rest of the family, especially when he became combative in the mornings.

Reluctant to place her uncle in an institution, Hinchcliffe has arranged for a professional caregiver to help him get ready each weekday morning. However, this arrangement puts financial strain on the family and she often works double shifts to make ends meet. And Hinchcliffe has to use vacation time when the caregiver is sick in order to take care of her uncle. She has trouble fitting in fun activities for the family amid the heavy burden of care.

Profiled in a report advocating for better support for caregivers in the UK, Hinchcliffe's experience illustrates that even a robust public system like the United Kingdom's can do a better job supporting health caregivers and decision makers.[27] Unlike many other countries, the UK does provide cash benefits to both a caregiver and care recipient—however, the restrictions to receiving such benefits are quite stringent and, according to the OECD, only one in ten caregivers received an allowance in 2008. Because the allowance is given to those with low income, the policy incentivizes caregivers to reduce their work hours in order to qualify for the benefit.

PART TWO: WOMEN'S HEALTHCARE NEEDS

5

The Time Famine

Nearly everyone in the modern world is short of time, and the pressures on working mothers are notorious. But what may surprise healthcare professionals is how widespread and severe the time shortage is, how much it is impacting women's health, and how little the industry is doing to address it. Addressing this time famine would likely improve women's health and win loyal customers. Our research shows that, across markets, 62 percent of women who think they should do much more about their health lack the time to do so. The specifics depend on lifestyle—not life stage—and point to time-saving services women would choose if given the option.

Among working mothers who think they should do more for their health, 78 percent say "lack of time" is an obstacle. Startlingly for those unused to a gender lens, 73 percent of working women *without kids* also say that time constraints keep them from taking care of their health as they should. Sixty-four percent of working moms with children over the age of eighteen say the same.

Figure 5.1
WOMEN WHO CITE TIME AS THE REASON THEY DON'T DO WHAT THEY THINK
THEY SHOULD DO TO STAY HEALTHY
(All markets)

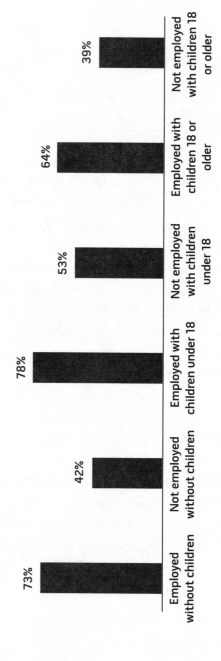

Stay-at-home moms would also be grateful for time-saving health solutions. More than half—53 percent—who say they should be doing more for their own health see time as an obstacle, as do 42 percent of stay-at-home women who don't have children. In addition to suffering from this time famine, stay-at-home mothers cite money as a big reason why they don't do what they know they should to stay healthy.

A PROBLEM FOR ALL INCOME LEVELS

The 24/7 nature of high-powered careers coupled with women's ongoing responsibility for the "second shift" (caring for children, tending the home) leaves professional women short of time for their own health. Of women in the US top household income bracket who say they aren't doing what they should to keep up with their health, 81 percent say they experience time famine.

The story of Lisa, a partner at a management consulting firm, is all too common. After three weeks with a sore throat, she took herself to an emergency room while on a business trip to Portland, OR. The ER physician told her that she was one step away from a life-threatening infection. "You're a grown woman, running a fever, you have chills, you should know better than to wait three weeks to see a doctor!" he tells Lisa.

Because Lisa, even though she has no children, is still a chief medical officer.

"I'm busy working, my husband is a diabetic and I'm helping him with that, and I'm looking after my extended family. My health comes last," she says. She also spends a lot of time and energy making healthcare decisions for her three siblings, who do have kids. She often helps pay for their healthcare too. "I am responding to a lot of reach-outs," she says. "I'm doing health research for my nieces and nephews when my sister doesn't have time. I'm trying to figure out the best way to help given my own responsibilities and commitments with my husband and my career. I simply don't have time to invest in myself."

Little wonder that, given the strain of delivering on multiple fronts, women are twice as likely as men to suffer from anxiety, with depression frequently co-occurring.[28]

On the other end of the income spectrum, as Jodi Kantor reported in "Working Anything but 9 to 5" in *The New York Times,* the unpredictable nature of work in the service economy and the need to take on multiple jobs can leave low-income women in the US with very little time for the roles they play at home.[29] Seventy-one percent of those who say they're not doing what they should to stay healthy also told us that they experience time famine. The double whammy? As 83 percent of working women in the bottom household income bracket of our US survey respondents indicated, they lack the money to pay for services that could potentially fill in the time gap.

Figure 5.2
WHY WOMEN DON'T DO WHAT THEY SAY THEY
SHOULD DO TO STAY HEALTHY: TIME VS. MONEY
(US employed women)

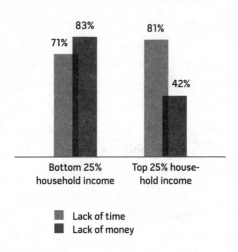

Male healthcare executives who lack training and experience in using a gender lens often miss how women, whether rich or poor, working or not working, mothers or not, take on enormous time pressures related to healthcare and leave themselves for last.

"Women are constantly putting others before themselves," says Christina Meringolo, a healthcare expert who has researched the female market for pharmaceutical companies. According to her qualitative research, at every age and stage, no matter whom they cared for or what their relationship was with the healthcare industry, "time was an extremely precious resource for women."

WHAT WOMEN WANT

Consider Sarah,* fifty, a divorced woman without kids who is a customer service manager for a major telephone conferencing company in Missouri. When her twin brother committed suicide, Sarah became her seventy-nine-year-old mother's CMO. "I'm the only family member in town," she says. "I was calling her three times a day, prepping her pillbox every week, and visiting often to check in on her health."

Then Sarah's mother fell and broke her hip, multiplying Sarah's responsibilities as health proxy. Her mother required multiple surgeries, which triggered delirium. Sarah took an emergency leave from work to be with her mother in the hospital and to find a rehabilitation facility. The initial facility in which her mother was placed struck Sarah as woefully inadequate, since the staff made many mistakes in her mother's regimens and care. Now Sarah is trying to determine whether her mother can return home with a full-time health aide or move into an assisted living facility. "I feel lucky to have a supportive boss who stretched my leave to the limit, but he is getting firmer about needing me to work a full week," she says.

Sarah's own health needs have also increased. She entered therapy just after her brother's suicide and went onto antidepressants for a while, but she's no longer in therapy or taking medication. She'd love to have more time to spend with friends, exercise, and relax, but right now she can barely juggle her work and her mother's care, let alone pay attention to her own well-being. "I'm near the end of my rope," Sarah says. "It's just so much to handle, and I'm losing myself in the process."

As Sarah's experience makes clear, the first casualty to time famine is often the CMO's emotional well-being. Only 37 percent of working women without kids actually undertake activities to manage stress.

HELPING WOMEN GET THEIR LIVES BACK

Physicians are well aware of time famine and its costs. Often serving as women's primary care physicians, the OB/GYNs interviewed for this study spoke frequently about how packed schedules made many patients ignore their own health.

"Sometimes a woman will come in to see me who hasn't had an annual appointment for twenty years," says the Cleveland Clinic OB/GYN Natalie Bowersox. "At first I am shocked, but then I think about my own life and how easy it might be to let that appointment slide."

When I heard Bowersox's words, they really hit home for me. I realized that, during the three years of my late husband's sickness, I hadn't gotten a mammogram or pap smear. That was especially unwise since my mother had breast cancer which, statistically, increases my own risk.

OB/GYN Shireen Jayne, who is affiliated with Froedtert and the Medical College of Wisconsin, hears about time famine regularly from her patients. "They want to get a prescription for a yeast or urinary tract infection over the phone, because they don't have time to come in," she says. She adds that it's a missed opportunity for the industry to help fight the time famine. "Healthcare organizations require that they visit the doctor in person, when I'd rather just prescribe it so that they can get a remedy as quickly as possible."

PRACTICAL IDEAS

Healthcare providers and industry specialists have shared insights that point to solutions. Kelly Barnes, leader of the US Health Industries practice at PwC, points out that as healthcare deductibles rise, and patients pay for more services out-of-pocket, treatment alternatives have emerged to provide fast, low-cost, convenient medical care at pharmacies and local clinics. That's pressuring all traditional healthcare industry players to provide greater time efficiency for patients and CMOs. "Now that decisions are more out-of-pocket and there's less of a hassle to provide insurance information for medical services, there's an opportunity to win over healthcare decision makers by providing convenience and saving them time," Barnes says.

Time-saving measures could include: evening office hours; nurses and doctors who make themselves available for consultations via online videoconferencing; and providers who email health regimens to CMOs and patients and allow them to make appointments online.

Tech start-ups are constantly developing new apps to save patients time in monitoring their blood pressure or other health indicators, or to ease communications between patients and health professionals.[30] Adopting any of these measures, Barnes says, would translate into a competitive advantage to the healthcare providers, pharmacies, and insurance companies that offer them. "What's stopping the companies from going there? Time, money, and risk-averse attitudes," Barnes says. "But they're missing enormous opportunities."

More ideas from healthcare professionals follow:

"How to become more consumer-focused, convenient, and more available? Have customer and patient reachout calls from seven p.m. to nine p.m. at night. Create an FAQ online, or email follow-up instructions—because if you give me a piece of paper at the doctors' office, chances are it's in a recycle bin somewhere."

—Kelly Barnes,
Leader of US Health Industries Practice, PwC

"We synchronize prescriptions monthly for families and provide a delivery service. So we're able to deliver all of their medications, for all generations, in one fell swoop each month."
—DJ Larson, Vice President of Marketing, Lehan Drugs

"We try to assign one caregiver in the family to administer medication to a patient to avoid too many people from getting involved or confused. It is actually more efficient that way."

—Regine Remy, RN, Lincoln Medical Center
and New York Presbyterian Hospital

"Being able to access a care provider without a face-to-face visit would help greatly. I want to solve my healthcare needs in a way that would allow me not to have to take time out of the day, or take my kids out of school, or arrange transport for my mom. Furthermore, being able to do that on Saturday, or at seven p.m., outside of usual business hours, would be ideal."

—Patti Harvey, Senior Vice President, Medicare Clinical
Operations and Population Care, Kaiser Foundation
Hospitals and Kaiser Foundation Health Plan, Inc.

6

The Trust Famine

Only 22 percent of women trust their insurance providers. A mere 17 percent of women trust their pharmaceutical companies. Less than half trust their pharmacists. While 65 percent do trust physicians, that's still an astonishingly low number for a professional with whom women are supposed to have an intimate relationship.

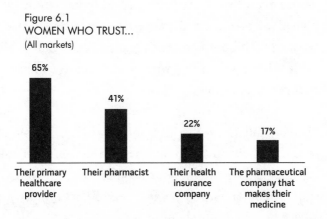

Figure 6.1
WOMEN WHO TRUST...
(All markets)

In retrospect, the problem was predictable. By excluding women from clinical trials, failing to diagnose them and give them effective remedies, inadequately researching gender differences in diseases and remedies, regularly ignoring input from caregivers and CMOs, and failing to ascertain women's preferences as consumers, the industry has lost women's faith.

Solutions are possible. Even pharmaceutical companies, further removed from the end user, have many opportunities to help their immediate customers—doctors, insurers, hospital administrators, and pharmacists—to build trusting, lasting relationships with patients and family CMOs. It will take work, and the first step is to understand the problem.

A TYPICAL STORY

Throughout her thirties, Barbara* paid little attention to healthcare. She shared her medical history with her doctor and got regular health screenings; she kept an eye on a few hereditary health issues in her family like high blood pressure and diabetes. On the whole, she felt satisfied with both her health and her care. But in her forties, her relationship with the healthcare industry changed dramatically.

"I'm now ferocious," she says. "Every year, our birthday gift from our insurance provider is a blood test. If it shows that I have low iron, I won't just call my doctor. I research it heavily online. Half the time, I skip the doctor entirely because then I'd have to pay for advice I could just find online myself."

Why the dramatic shift? At thirty-eight, Barbara decided to start a family. Single at the time, she adopted Andre,* a boy who had already lived in more than eight foster homes by the time he turned five and met Barbara. Diagnosed with ADHD, he began taking Concerta. And his reaction—"an hour after taking the medication, he was like a zombie for another couple of hours"—so alarmed Barbara that she asked his pediatrician to prescribe an alternative.

The doctor's response, when she asked if a drug like Adderall might work better, was less than reassuring. "Okay, do you want to try that instead?" he asked Barbara. She'd hoped for more of a collaboration. "I mean, I thought the whole point was for him to advise me," she recalls. "He was just abdicating responsibility."

Barbara convinced the pediatrician to investigate Adderall further, and to discuss Andre's case with colleagues who had tried the drug on their own patients; eventually they decided not to put Andre on Adderall but instead to change the Concerta dosage, which worked. "But in the interim, we were playing with a cocktail of drugs," says Barbara. "I hated to be just trying things on him. It was incredibly frustrating to have to push so hard for support from the pediatrician."

This experience has left Barbara leery of the entire system when it comes to Andre's care, which goes beyond medical treatment. So she's stepped up her own role as CMO. When Andre decided to go off of his ADHD medication a couple of years ago, she connected him with a therapist who helps him control his anger and tune up his emotional intelligence. Since the local school system tests Andre periodically to assess whether he belongs in special education classes, she uses her vacation time to accompany him.

Now married, Barbara pushes her husband to take on healthier habits, too. She's joined an insurance coverage program that charges a premium for members who smoke (as her husband does) in an effort—so far unsuccessful, and therefore expensive—to provide an incentive for him to quit. She also gets heavily involved in healthcare decision-making for her parents, and calls her mother's doctors before and after appointments. If a friend is diagnosed with a serious illness, Barbara asks her about her regimen, and helps her with research. She keeps track of her findings with an app on her iPad that stores text and multimedia files. "I will record anything, take notes, and attach photos," she says.

Barbara's approach to her role as CMO of her family is incredibly time-consuming and insomnia-inducing. While grateful that her employer has supported her need to balance career and family care, she has turned down several promotions over the years. She is constantly filling in for gaps she discovers in her family's healthcare—from diagnosis, to medical record-keeping, to making appointments, to researching new medical innovations. It takes a lot for Barbara to sign off on a prescription or regimen recommendation from a healthcare professional for anyone in her circle.

"The way our system is set up now, everyone can get tricked by studies and marketing from pharmaceutical companies, even doctors," Barbara says. "Let's face it, they get visits from salespeople, who win the doctors' trust, and then the doctors don't have time to dig into the research that the sales representative presents."

IGNORED IN CLINICAL TRIALS

Women have long been excluded from clinical trials and studied less closely than men. The decision probably seemed reasonable to all or mostly-male executive teams: it requires extra money and effort to include women, whose presence also increases variability in data. Pregnant women add yet another layer of cost and difficulty.

Until 1988, clinical trials of new drugs were conducted on predominantly male subjects, though women consumed 80 percent of the pharmaceuticals in the US at the time. It wasn't until 1994 that the FDA formed the Office of Women's Health (OWH). The office's mission is to "protect and advance the health of women through policy, science, and outreach"— including "advocating for women in clinical trials and for sex, gender, and subpopulation analyses."

According to the OWH, women have nearly double the risk of developing an adverse drug reaction as men, but in 2001, two-thirds of trials still excluded women. While 91 percent of studies found evidence that gender made a difference in the way drugs were metabolized or in the occurrence of adverse reactions, scientists failed to analyze results.[31] As a result of this omission, there's little understanding about potential differences between male and female responses to medicines. "The research on medications has not been sampling women or minorities as much as it should," says Teri Aronowitz, a PhD and board-certified family nurse practitioner who studies primary care and sexual health. "We don't have nearly enough knowledge about whether a given product will work the same on a woman as it would on a man, or on an African American woman versus a white male."

This norm is changing—the National Institute of Health is requiring more inclusion of female animals in preclinical studies—but the depth of the impact remains to be seen.[32] "Will it change how science is done? It should, but there's still a question if it will," says Virginia M. Miller, MD, director of the Women's Health Research Center and Specialized Center of Research on Sex Differences at the Mayo Clinic. "There aren't clear guidelines on how the new policies will be implemented and tracked, and whether there is a consequence for not complying with the new regulations."

Medical professionals are just beginning to understand sex differences in heart disease, according to physicians we interviewed. "When I was in medical school, there was no instruction about women and heart disease. The common wisdom was that they didn't really get heart attacks, or they were really elderly when they did," said Sharonne N. Hayes, MD, a cardiologist at the Mayo Clinic in Rochester, Minnesota, who founded Mayo's Women's Heart Clinic. "But that wasn't based on hard research—outside of 'bikini medicine,' breasts and reproductive health, the research on women just wasn't there."

Much progress has been made in caring for women's hearts, Hayes acknowledges, especially important since heart disease is their number one killer. Researchers now know that there are important differences between women and men when it comes to cardiovascular disease, ranging from genetics, to risk factors, to symptoms and how best to make diagnoses and recommend treatment. But Hayes says medicine still doesn't fully understand why heart disease manifests itself so differently between men and women. Sex and gender-specific research is also lacking in many other medical conditions.

There is still a lot of work to be done. In 2015, a bipartisan bill called the Research for All Act, which would mandate that clinical drug trials for fast-tracked drugs take safety into account for both men and women, was introduced to the House. "One sex should not be excluded from testing when it could mean the difference between effective treatment and harm to health," Congresswoman Cynthia Lummis said.[33]

As of the time of this book's publication, the Research for All Act hasn't gotten out of committee.[34]

IGNORED IN THE EXAM ROOM

"I've had bladder problems my whole life, and one time I asked my OB/GYN whether I might be allergic to my menstrual pads," says Linda,* a CEO of a boutique advertising agency. "She responded, 'Why are you wearing those every day?' I had never thought about it as abnormal, but of course, it was for urinary leaking." Linda's doctor recommended she try a different brand of menstrual pad. He didn't prescribe anything; he didn't send Linda to a urologist. "For me, it was an 'aha!' moment, so I went to the urologist myself and now I have a remedy for the problem," Linda says. "But it wasn't based on my OB/GYN's recommendation."

Linda isn't the first woman to need to take charge of her own care. According to broad research of the female healthcare consumer market conducted by Sandra,* a pharmaceutical executive, women ages forty-five to sixty-four struggle with a host of issues for which they find little guidance from the healthcare system, including urinary issues. Fully 26 percent of women experience urinary symptoms, the company found, but the majority fail to get a diagnosis. Those who are diagnosed often fail to get adequate treatment. On average, their research showed that women present their symptoms eight times to their doctors before receiving treatment. Why? Because these are complex issues, Sandra says, that often require longer, probing conversations with providers during time-constrained appointments that may be used to address multiple conditions.

Sandra decided to tackle the challenge of underdiagnosis and undertreatment, since so many women experience it. While her work may have increased prescription rates of her company's medicines that treat underdiagnosed conditions like urinary incontinence, her main objective was to raise awareness of this issue.

Sandra and her team approached leaders inside and outside of the company, educating them on her research and seeking a solution to help reduce the number of times a woman would have to bring up symptoms to her doctor before receiving diagnosis and any warranted treatment. In order to provide a solution women could trust, Sandra created a partnership with highly respected medical organizations to solidify a set of screening questions for overactive bladder and other conditions that could live in the electronic medical record. She partnered with some of the world's largest medical practices to implement pilot programs.

"Because of quality measures, these systems now have incentives to improve satisfaction rates because it affects their bottom line. It also affects their practice efficiency, if their patients are coming back eight times due to a single issue," Sandra says. By giving doctors systemized tools to diagnose and recommend treatment if necessary, she hypothesized that prescriptions of various medications to treat urinary incontinence would likely increase.

Sandra gained traction externally, working with medical groups to refine the screening tools and include them in electronic medical records. These partners expanded the screenings to include other conditions for which women are underdiagnosed, like fibromyalgia.

Sandra also fought hard for internal support at her company, using the external collaborations as leverage and to set aggressive deadlines. She leveraged the internal executive sponsor of the project, using his name regularly to demonstrate institutional backing. She would meet with colleagues before and after presentations to gain their buy-in one-on-one. "It was enormously time-consuming, but I was deeply passionate about this," Sandra says. The pilot was successfully deployed in 2013, and she developed an aggressive expansion plan.

Then, Sandra and her executive sponsor were both transferred to new roles. "It's very challenging to do things that buck the system unless you have an enormous amount of sponsorship at the very top levels," she says. After she was transferred, her program continued, but only with a smaller staff and budget. The aggressive expansion is looking unlikely, and there isn't the bandwidth to collect the impact metrics Sandra would like to see. Prescription rates of her company's overactive bladder and fibromyalgia medicines went up after these new screenings were deployed at the medical practices in the program, but she is pessimistic that it will be scaled up further.

"It's a real shame," she says, "because I found an area of huge opportunity. I kept trying to get my colleagues to get past their unconscious biases about 'women's health' and see the unquestionable market opportunity I was presenting."

Sandra's dogged pursuit of better urinary incontinence diagnosis for women reveals a major obstacle the industry faces in building trust with women: women are aware that they're underdiagnosed. This is particularly true in the case of mental health.

In our survey, 32 percent of working moms, 23 percent of stay-at-home moms, and 42 percent of working women without kids report having symptoms consistent with anxiety issues, but haven't been diagnosed by their doctors. A majority (52 percent) of working women without kids who report symptoms of social anxiety disorders haven't been diagnosed by their doctors as having anxiety. Having mental health issues go unacknowledged by medical health professionals contributes to women's mistrust of the industry.

Figure 6.2
WOMEN WHO SELF-REPORT A HEALTH ISSUE THAT REMAINS
UNDIAGNOSED BY A PHYSICIAN

Women who self-report having...	% who have not been diagnosed by a doctor
Obsessive compulsive disorder	43%
Anxiety	35%
Social anxiety disorder	34%
Insomnia	33%
Panic disorder	21%
Depression	20%
Post-traumatic stress disorder	17%

STAY AT HOME MOMS ARE ESPECIALLY SKEPTICAL

As a child suffering from renal tubular acidosis, Daniel experienced delayed speech and other developmental delays, along with depression and stunted growth. His stay-at-home mother and caregiver, Susan Medansky, acted as his advocate from the moment he was diagnosed, enrolling him in Illinois's free developmental therapies for children under the age of three.

When his growth rate fell far below age-appropriate benchmarks, his pediatrician suggested he take Nutropin, a Genentech hormone therapy that would stimulate his growth. But the family's insurance didn't cover Nutropin, and on her then-husband's $65,000 annual salary, Medansky couldn't afford the treatment's out-of-pocket cost. "I considered taking on a job myself to cover the cost of the therapy," she says, "but my son needed so much attention I didn't see how I could leave him."

The pediatrician proved unhelpful—when Medansky asked him for alternatives to paying out-of-pocket for Nutropin, he offered no solutions. "I still get angry that pharmaceutical companies make so much profit because of the cost of drugs," Medansky says. "Some drugs are expensive to produce. But with others, they just want to make a profit. I think they gouge people sometimes."

Stay-at-home mothers are especially unlikely to trust the healthcare industry: only 12 percent of them trust insurance providers, and only 12 percent trust pharmaceutical companies. Numbers among stay-at-home women without kids are similar. While trust in the industry is low across the board among women, it's higher among working mothers (see figure 6.3). Stay-at-home mothers also rarely trust information from major brands; just 13 percent of them say that affiliation with a major brand makes a source of healthcare information trustworthy.

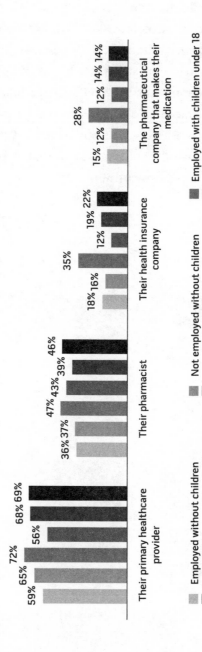

Figure 6.3
WOMEN WHO TRUST...
(All markets)

Why do stay-at-home moms distrust the industry? Perhaps because the industry shows less trust in them. For example, we asked stay-at-home mothers what assumptions their doctors make about them. Just 22 percent of them have the sense that their doctors think they understand the doctor's advice. With working mothers, the number jumps to 31 percent, and it rises even higher among empty nesters, whether they work or not.

Figure 6.4
WOMEN WHO REPORT THAT THEIR PRIMARY
HEALTHCARE PROVIDER ASSUMES...
(All markets)

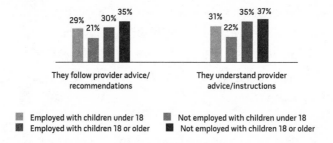

They follow provider advice/recommendations — 29% 21% 30% 35%

They understand provider advice/instructions — 31% 22% 35% 37%

▨ Employed with children under 18   ▨ Not employed with children under 18
■ Employed with children 18 or older   ■ Not employed with children 18 or older

"As a stay-at-home mom, I just don't get the respect I deserve from my son's pediatrician," said one respondent in a focus group. "This doctor doesn't listen to me, ignores the online research I spent hours gathering—it's incredibly frustrating."

In addition, stay-at-home mothers surviving on one income are often more concerned about financial constraints in healthcare. As we saw with the time famine in Chapter Five, many ignore their own health because of lack of money. Hence, the high cost of certain drugs hits closer to home for them than for others.

HOW TO EARN WOMEN'S TRUST

The industry can take several steps to win women's trust. First, it has to make transparent the number of women who participate in clinical trials and include more women in order to fully understand how a medicine affects women and men differently.

"There's always room to do everything better. We can have more women involved in clinical trials. It can be more difficult to recruit women to participate. In part due to pregnancy and hormonal cycles, there are particular challenges for women as we're trying to improve diversity in clinical trials. But the recruitment is absolutely important, because you want the data to reflect differences there may be in women," says Roslyn F. Schneider, MD, Global Patient Affairs lead at Pfizer. "We have to be very transparent about the strength of the data in clinical trials."

Pharmaceutical companies can also work with providers to improve diagnosis rates for women. Like Sandra's employer, a growing number of pharmaceutical companies are aware of underdiagnosis in overactive bladder and urinary incontinence.

"Women have developed enormous coping strategies when it comes to overactive bladder. When you have a meaningful product available, it can be enormously empowering and freeing to say, 'You don't have to cope with this!'" says Karen Scollick, vice president for global marketing, innovation, and marketing services at Merck and Co. "The more we can identify conditions like that for women, the more we can help them and open up new spaces for our companies." Given the survey findings, emotional health and heart disease issues can be added to that list for women.

Finally, pharmaceutical companies can provide better alternatives for CMOs like Susan Medansky, who have trouble affording their remedies. Determined to get her son the medicine he needed, Medansky shared her frustration with friends and family. Finally, an acquaintance at a playgroup mentioned that some pharmaceutical companies offered assistance for families with limited insurance and income.

Medansky researched Genentech and, to her relief, discovered they offered such a program. She applied, qualified, and for the following year received monthly supplies and injections for her son. Genentech even sent special coolers and ice packs to keep the Nutropin refrigerated when the family traveled.

This program spared Medansky thousands of dollars in treatment expenses each month, and allowed her son to cross off his list of developmental challenges the most significant and socially penalizing: small stature. "Given the other challenges he faced, I simply couldn't consider ignoring this one, which could be helped so dramatically," Medansky says. Today, Daniel is a senior in high school and looking forward to attending college.

Medansky takes immense pride in his progress. "I just wish the process of finding out about this assistance and applying for it had been more transparent and easier to navigate," she says. In other interviews, we heard many similar calls for a more navigable system of existing assistance programs from pharmaceutical companies.

As they begin to court consumers for a wider array of health and clinical services, US pharmacies are starting to build trust with women. Take CVS's recent decision to stop selling tobacco products in its stores, a point of pride for Helena B. Foulkes, executive vice president of CVS Health and president of CVS/pharmacy.

For years, as Foulkes worked to expand CVS's partnerships with hospital systems, health insurance providers and other health companies, her meetings hit turbulence when potential partners raised concerns about CVS's $200 billion in annual revenues from the sales of tobacco products. CVS's continued sales of these products also became a point of disengagement for the company's employees.

Foulkes spoke at an *Economist* conference two weeks after the tobacco products were pulled from CVS shelves. She raved about the trust the company's decision had already created with its stakeholders. "I think what's been really exciting is the energy this decision has really unleashed, both among people who use our stores—that response has been unbelievable—but also the pride among our more than two hundred thousand employees that work across the company," she said. "They feel very, very proud that the company would make a decision like this. What it really represents for us is the marriage of all the things we do to help patients."[35]

A holistic vision of CVS as a healthcare company—and how that alters the company's business model and the way it connects with stakeholders—shows CVS is taking trust into consideration as it looks to expand its role in the healthcare industry. These actions may have helped CVS Health vault eighteen spots forward on *Fortune Magazine*'s ranking of the World's Most Admired Companies, reaching number twenty-seven in 2016.[36]

PRACTICAL IDEA: HEALTHCARE ADVISOR

To generate ideas to help the healthcare industry meet women's needs, I convened executives from pharmaceutical, insurance, consulting, and healthcare marketing firms to think about solutions that would better tap the power of the purse in healthcare, while also meeting one or more of the famines that women face. At a full-day Innovation Lab, facilitated by CTI, the executives split up into teams charged with fleshing out transformational ideas. One team focused on a new professional service—healthcare advice—that could build trust between different parts of the healthcare system. Here's how team presenter Dan Movens, senior vice president and general manager at Cardinal Health, described a "healthcare advisor":

"Similar to a financial advisor, a healthcare advisor could serve as an independent, professional, trusted partner for the CMO of a household. At the beginning of a relationship, this healthcare advisor would administer a diagnostic to understand the client's 'health profile.' Then, the advisor can help the patient by navigating the patient's care and the care of family members, making decisions that best fit their lifestyle and preferences, tracking health maintenance needs, finding doctors, navigating insurance claims, and answering other questions that arise. This new role presents an enormous opportunity for entrepreneurs as healthcare moves to a consumer-focused model. Given women's hunger for trusted relationships and information when it comes to healthcare, as well as limits on their time to make decisions, a trusted partner can help them navigate the complex healthcare landscape and sit with them at the center of care.

"Given the dearth of trust in healthcare, an advisor has an enormous opportunity to serve as a bridge between industry and the CMO. Women of all ages, cultures, and backgrounds can collaborate with this advisor over decades to find the health solutions they seek."

7

The Knowledge Famine

Women are hungry for information, but they're not getting it. Seventy-three percent of women say that it's very important to them to be knowledgeable about keeping themselves and their loved ones healthy, according to our research. Women don't want to delegate their CMO responsibilities.

Sixty-five percent of women say they trust their doctors, but given the time famine—for patients and physicians—women have to seek information elsewhere. Since they don't trust the industry, they don't trust the information that companies provide. Instead they go online, and they ask their friends and families. They collect more opinion than fact, or packets of information without context tailored to their own situation and preferences. Yet they know this ad hoc approach falls short: even though 53 percent of women think they can get the best healthcare information from the Internet, only 31 percent of these women trust the information they get online.

Figure 7.1
WOMEN AND INTERNET HEALTH RESOURCES

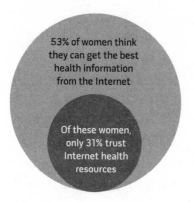

The healthcare industry can gain women's trust and loyalty if it helps them become more health literate, through direct or indirect channels.

Anne Klibanski, neuroendocrinologist and chief academic officer at Massachusetts hospital system Partners HealthCare, has interviewed many women to understand the kind of knowledge they seek, and whether they feel underinformed about health. It's now part of a larger effort to educate patients about research opportunities that are relevant to their health, which will be integrated into the hospitals' online information and electronic medical records so that they are more user-friendly for patients and for CMOs. Her findings so far? "It's not coordinated," Klibanski says. "You have so many choices. We need to tailor the choices to the patient and to a family, and make the information simpler to obtain and navigate. Right now, with an overwhelming assortment of things that no one can judge, it's very difficult for individual women to discern trustworthy information about their health."

HISPANIC WOMEN FEEL THE FAMINE

Hispanic women in the US are unlikely even to trust their physicians' information. Instead, they look elsewhere to fill in for the doctor, and that can provide an opportunity for healthcare or other kinds of companies. Media company Univision, for example, is looking to become a trusted source of health information for Hispanics. "As a trusted pillar of our community, Univision is in a unique position to reach Hispanics," says Jorge Daboub, senior vice president of business development at Univision, which began partnering with Kaiser Family Foundation on AIDS awareness decades ago. Univision has developed live programs, television advertising, public service announcements, and online platforms to educate viewers about health.

Figure 7.2
WOMEN WHO SAY THEY CAN GET THE BEST INFORMATION ABOUT KEEPING THEMSELVES AND THEIR LOVED ONES HEALTHY FROM THEIR PRIMARY HEALTHCARE PROVIDER (US)

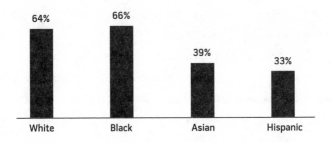

White	Black	Asian	Hispanic
64%	66%	39%	33%

Having studied viewers' health outlooks and habits, Daboub can explain why Hispanics feel excluded from traditional sources of information. "Only three percent of US doctors are Hispanic," he says. "More importantly, though, few physicians are culturally sensitive to Hispanic patients and what they're looking for. Hispanic patients are very familial, very community-oriented; and women are absolutely the authority figures in their families when it comes to health."

When a Hispanic patient visits a doctor, Daboub explains, the patient is generally accompanied by a female family member who expects to be part of the decision-making process. Many doctors, working under severe time constraints, find this arrangement burdensome and inefficient—an attitude that comes through in their patient interactions. "Very nuanced changes in their patient interactions could help those patients digest the information better," Daboub says.

Because doctors are so highly respected in Hispanic countries, he adds, Hispanic patients may feel shy about starting a dialogue. They also may hesitate to ask follow-up questions, so their risk of not adhering to prescribed regimens grows. "Doctors here need to find better ways to reinforce the health regimens they are recommending," Daboub says.

To some degree, the industry is aware of these inconsistencies in healthcare delivery, and has taken steps to address them. For example, Pfizer partners with Venus Ginés, a breast cancer survivor who trains *promotores*—community health workers certified to perform health assessments and screenings—to fill in gaps in health services in Latino communities. "It's not enough to translate brochures into Spanish," she says. "We learn differently. We rely more on stories and visuals to process information."

Ginés has been working with Pfizer as well as other organizations to develop information that speaks to Latinos, from producing *novelita* comic books that educate readers about health risks to materials that educate promotores about the financial assistance programs available at Pfizer and other companies. Still, Ginés says, her work cannot address all of the ways the system ignores Latinos.

"There is two percent Latino enrollment in clinical trials. That's pathetic," she says. "I worked with a pharmaceutical company and consulting company in New Mexico, and I was constantly telling them to speak directly with Latinas for their research. They're not getting out into the community, so they make erroneous assumptions. Then they produce a stick-figure diagram, or a direct English-to-Spanish translation that fails to communicate effectively with Latinos."

LIMITED HEALTH LITERACY

Latinas aren't the only women whom the industry has failed. Most women in our survey demonstrate limited health literacy. We asked respondents to report how knowledgeable they think they are about health and then gave them a health literacy quiz to test their actual knowledge. Forty percent of all women say they are knowledgeable; about the same amount, 43 percent, indeed demonstrated literacy in our quiz. Among Hispanic women in the US, 62 percent say they are knowledgeable, while only 39 percent passed our literacy quiz.[†]

Figure 7.3
PERCEIVED HEALTH KNOWLEDGE VS. TESTED LITERACY

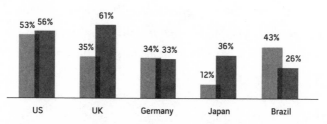

US   UK   Germany   Japan   Brazil

■ Women who say they are knowledgable about keeping themselves and their loved ones healthy
■ Women who pass our health literacy quiz[†]

Across countries, working mothers are unlikely to pass the literacy quiz—only 38 percent of working mothers passed—but are quite likely to say they are knowledgeable (53 percent report they feel knowledgeable). Given the finding that working mothers are also likely to see the Internet as their best available source of information (51 percent), it would appear that women are justified in their distrust of the web: it simply cannot supplant healthcare professionals in helping women understand medical issues, diagnose illnesses, or seek appropriate treatment options.

---

† With a score of 17/19 or above

Figure 7.4
PERCEIVED HEALTH KNOWLEDGE VS. TESTED LITERACY
(All markets)

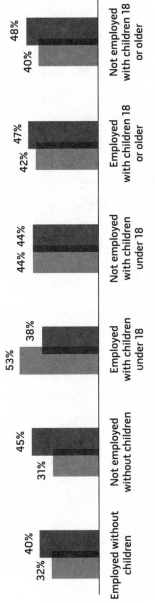

Women who say they are knowledgable about keeping themselves and their loved ones healthy
Women who pass our health literacy quiz

Online-sourced information may even undermine women in their quest for wellness. Many of the physicians we interviewed said "Dr. Google" can give patients and decision makers a false sense of certainty about their health. "It varies from patient to patient, but with the Internet, many patients are extremely well-informed before they walk in the door," says OB/GYN Shireen Jayne. "They've already Googled their bladder problem, their hysterectomy, or whatever, and they're certain they know the cause of their symptoms. I welcome their curiosity, but then I need to take a moment and re-educate them as to why they made the right or wrong assessment based on online information."

IMPLICATIONS FOR THE INDUSTRY

Women know they aren't health experts. Yet in their roles as decision makers for others, they want to know more—but 53 percent lack a trustworthy information source. High levels of stress related to making healthcare decisions contributes to women's hunger for information and, simultaneously, to their lack of knowledge. "Women always think there is more to learn. When they are under stress, they ask questions," says John Gray, author of *Men Are from Mars, Women Are from Venus* and other books exploring gender differences that persist in contemporary society. "To men, asking questions is a sign of incompetence, and incompetence is failure."

Gray has examined these gender tendencies in the context of healthcare, and found that men are far more willing than women are to delegate responsibilities for healthcare decision-making. Women, he found, eagerly collaborate with doctors and other healthcare professionals, and approach health challenges as a research project. Ninety percent of the time, he says, women think they're asking the right number of questions. On the other hand, he says, men are just as likely to think women ask too many questions.

In interviews we conducted, doctors and pharmacists often shared similar observations about male and female patients—that women tend to ask more questions, that they attend appointments more frequently, and that they second-guess doctor recommendations more often. DJ Larson, vice president of marketing for the independent pharmacy Lehan Drugs in DeKalb, Illinois, says he sees a deep hunger for trusted information among women.

"When men come to us, they're not shopping. They're buying," Larson says. "A female patient, on the other hand, generally has a lot more questions for us and wants to understand the reasoning behind taking a drug. Even though it has already been prescribed by a doctor, she is likely to still be considering whether to take it or not—and whether an over-the-counter remedy might also work. She's asking questions, looking for next steps."

Klibanski sees that research instinct among patients at Partners HealthCare hospital system, as well. "We have a group of patients willing to speak to others about their disease in online forums," she says. "The great majority of patients who take us up on that offer to connect with others are women. They want that personal accessibility."

In interviews, many executives at pharmaceutical companies shared a common frustration: given the extensive research they conduct in the design, development, and marketing of medicines, they have rich information to share with providers and patients. Yet because they operate in a highly regulated industry and lack trusting relationships with consumers, they are unable to turn their own websites and sales forces into trusted sources of information for providers, patients, and decision makers.

The industry could meet the knowledge famine in a few ways. First, it could train physicians and its own consumer-facing staff to be aware of women's inquisitive nature and their desire to be partners in healthcare research and decision-making. Next, it could introduce women to professionals who can serve as ongoing resources of information—for example, Lehan Drugs posts pictures and bios of all of its pharmacists online so that patients can put a face to a name before coming into the store. Finally, as Klibanski suggests, it could collaborate with other stakeholders to create more coordinated online sources of information.

These sources would provide many answers under a single umbrella, curated with the help of independent partners—in academia, for example—whom women trust. With the stamp of a trusted independent partner, pharmaceutical companies could find a platform for some of their most important findings for patients.

PRACTICAL IDEA: COMPREHENSIVE ONLINE PLATFORM

At the same Innovation Lab that generated the idea of a "professional healthcare advisor" explored in Chapter Six, another team developed the idea for a new online platform that would deliver trusted health information to women. Here's how team presenter Sandra Humbles, vice president of Global Education Solutions at Johnson & Johnson, described her vision for the platform:

"This trusted website would provide unbiased information about health and disease, forums with other patients and CMOs, and reviews of potential products and services in a simple, easy-to-read format. This platform would be a collaboration of tech start-ups, trusted healthcare associations, medical providers and health systems, pharmaceutical companies, and others. It could even connect to electronic medical records, providing a one-stop shop for information, discussion with peers, personal data, and ways to set up doctors' appointments for themselves and others. It must be curated carefully, and provide monitored forums, so women can connect to others with similar concerns while maintaining civil discourse. At the launch of the site, it can also feature high-level celebrity endorsements—think Oprah—to gain public trust. Since women go online first for health information, this solution would give them a better coordinated resource that could guide their conversations with their physicians and peers. We could start very targeted, focusing on women's heart health, and expand from there."

PART THREE: SOLUTIONS

8

Building New Relationships

Healthcare professionals who work directly with women patients and CMOs have to adopt behaviors that build trust and satisfy their core consumers' needs. To help companies and professionals understand what trust and satisfaction would mean for women, our survey asked women to select, from a long list, those behaviors exhibited by their healthcare professionals. Then the survey asked whether they trust (and are satisfied with) those professionals. We then correlated these two questions to identify which behaviors garner the most trust and satisfaction among female patients and consumers by sector. The results were filtered by geography, generation, income, and lifestyle to better understand what various female market segments seek from the healthcare industry. For the behaviors, see the illustration on the next page.

BEHAVIORS
THAT WIN WITH WOMEN

PHARMACISTS WHO...

- Provide them with the information they need to make decisions
- Ask and listen to their concerns/questions
- Discuss pharmaceutical options and alternatives
- Save them time

DOCTORS WHO...

- Report test results in an understandable way
- Discuss preventative care and proactively manage their health
- Ask and listen to their concerns/questions
- Provide them with the information they need to make decisions

HEALTH INSURANCE COMPANIES THAT...

- Provide coverage for doctors they trust
- Make preventative care affordable
- Make it easy to find a doctor in network
- Provide easy, friendly, and informative customer service

PHARMACEUTICAL COMPANIES THAT...

- Provide them clear information along with their prescription to help them understand risks and side effects
- Provide gender- and ethnic-specific drug recommendations
- Provide comprehensive information about their products on their website
- Make a person available by phone 24/7 to answer questions or concerns about their prescription

BECOMING A TRUSTED PRIMARY CARE PROVIDER

Building relationships with patients gets harder for doctors as their time in the exam room is increasingly constrained. "But, there's always time to say something, so why not say the right thing?" asks Lynn O'Connor Vos, CEO of ghg | greyhealth group, a healthcare marketing agency. She thinks that the industry can help doctors do a far better job of connecting with patients, both to improve patients' understandings of diagnoses and treatment options and to enhance their own understandings of the patients.

According to our research, women who trust and are satisfied with their primary healthcare providers find that their doctors are clear communicators and active listeners and that they proactively discuss preventative care. As in other areas of this research, women with different lifestyles identified different preferences. Understandably, working mothers who trust their doctors reported that their doctors provide clear, actionable recommendations on how to improve their health. Stay-at-home mothers reported having trusted doctors who treat their symptoms, demonstrate empathy and respect, provide more information, and create a safe space for patients to share their own concerns. Working women without children who trust their doctors say their doctors create a peer relationship, seek to understand their concerns and questions, and provide them with the information they need to make decisions.

Figure 8.1
WOMEN WHO REPORT THAT THEIR PRIMARY HEALTHCARE PROVIDER...
(All markets)

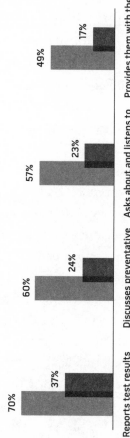

	Reports test results in an understand-able way[†]	Discusses preventative care and proactively manages their health[††]	Asks about and listens to their concerns/questions	Provides them with the information they need to make decisions
Women who are trusting and satisfied with their primary healthcare provider	70%	60%	57%	49%
Women who are NOT trusting and satisfied with their primary healthcare provider	37%	24%	23%	17%

▇ Women who are trusting and satisfied with their primary healthcare provider
▇ Women who are NOT trusting and satisfied with their primary healthcare provider

†   "Reports test results in an understandable way" is a net of "reports test results in an understandable way" and "explains test results/clinical information in a way I can understand"

††   "Discusses preventative care and proactively manages my health" is a net of "discusses preventive care measures" and "proactively manages my health by recommending screenings, tests, or procedures"

Lili Lustig is an example of what doctors can do, but her journey was a long one. For decades, she was a medical assistant and dental office manager, so she felt confident she could be a good health proxy for her mother, who suffers from scleroderma. But many interactions with her mother's doctors left her feeling frustrated and inadequate. "They would ignore me when I tried to communicate with them about my mother's medical history," she explains, "and they wouldn't discuss the rationale for her treatments. I had enough education that I knew some of what they were doing would not have successful results, and other procedures would, but they wouldn't listen to me."

After one particularly upsetting encounter, Lustig recalls turning to her husband and saying, "I could do a better job." He looked her in the eye, smiled, and said, "So? Go do it."

Lustig took his advice. Without a bachelor's degree—and with a two-year-old, a five-year-old, and a fifteen-year-old at home—she headed back to school to earn a bachelor's degree in biology and physiology. She applied to medical school and, at the age of forty-eight, uprooted her family from Arizona to begin her studies at the Virginia College of Osteopathic Medicine in Blacksburg, Virginia.

Upon graduation, Lustig moved her family again to enter a residency at the Cleveland Clinic in Ohio. Today, after a stint in an emergency medicine residency, Lustig is an attending physician in family medicine at a

Cleveland Clinic regional hospital. Many of her patients lack insurance, are unemployed, and have great medical needs. "Family medicine chose me," Lustig says. "I always wanted to know more about the patient than time allowed in the emergency room. So the program director came up to me and said, 'I really think you should try family medicine.'"

Lustig's experience as a healthcare proxy for her mother informed how she interacts with patients, who tend to have low health literacy. She tries to communicate with them respectfully while still educating them about the basics. "I use a lot of analogies with my patients," Lustig says. For example, she'll compare blood pressure to the pressure of water in a clogged garden hose—the pressure can cause the hose to burst. Because these explanations take up time that her appointment schedule rarely accommodates, Lustig asks patients to return so that she can monitor how they're doing with their prescription regimens, and to ensure that they understand her recommendations. Because the language on Cleveland Clinic's electronic medical health record can be too hard for them to understand, she often writes out clearer instructions.

If a male patient comes into her office with a female spouse or relative, Lustig takes pains to share her recommendations with both of them, as she knows her patient is more likely to adhere to regimens if that female relative feels included in his care. She's also gotten better adherence from her patients by providing them with clearer English translations of complicated information from pharmaceutical companies and insurance providers, translations that a member of her staff provides. "I am so driven to make a difference, because I understand their frustrations and desires to be taken seriously," Lustig says.

Lustig is a model for the industry in creating relationships with patients, caregivers, and CMOs to drive better health outcomes through increased adherence to prescribed regimens that both treat and prevent illness. She has the "point-of-pain" insight that providers need in order to diagnose and treat underserved market segments, and she has acquired, through personal experience, the empathy that sustains her commitment.

BECOMING A TRUSTED PHARMACEUTICAL COMPANY

As pharmaceutical companies connect ever more directly with consumers, it becomes imperative they understand which behaviors will help women trust them as healthcare partners. Trusted pharmaceutical companies that earn customer satisfaction, according to women across all five of the markets in our survey, provide clear information about risks and side effects in prescription inserts, gender- and ethnic-specific drug recommendations, comprehensive product information online, and 24/7 availability of customer service representatives.

Figure 8.2
WOMEN WHO REPORT THAT THE PHARMACEUTICAL COMPANY THAT
MAKES THEIR MEDICINE...
(All markets)

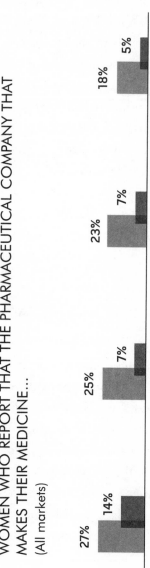

Provides clear informa-tion along with their prescription to help them understand the risks and side effects — 27% / 14%

Provides gender- and ethnic-specific drug recommendations — 25% / 7%

Provides comprehensive information about its products on its website — 23% / 7%

Makes a person available by phone 24/7 to answer questions or concerns about their prescription — 18% / 5%

Women who are trusting and satisfied with their pharmaceutical company
Women who are NOT trusting and satisfied with their pharmaceutical company

What might this look like in practice? Perhaps something like the BioScience division of Baxter International, Inc., headquartered in Deerfield, Illinois, which is working to become a trusted pharmaceutical partner among mothers of hemophilia patients. A disease carried genetically by women that almost always presents in men, hemophilia is a rare blood disorder in which the blood doesn't clot properly. Those with hemophilia risk damage especially to their joints from bleeding, particularly if treated inadequately over the long-term. Baxter makes an injectable drug that helps facilitate blood clotting, and is used as a preventative therapy for hemophilia patients. The dosage of the drug depends both on the individual patient and his risk of getting a cut or scrape.

Since the disease presents early in life, Baxter knows that it is patients' mothers who will oversee their choice of medication and adherence to it. "We spend a lot of time thinking about how we can enhance the experience of the caregiver," says Brian Goff, former president of hematology at Baxalta. "We consider how the medicine is delivered to these moms, the information they receive, and how they can customize the dose of the medication to the exact blood level necessary to help prevent bleeds in their sons based on the activities they're engaging in. To build trust, we aim to provide high quality treatments, consistency in product availability, and clear information and education."

As the firm is also aware of mothers' time constraints, Goff and his team are developing simple, technological tools that help caregivers quickly access information about hemophilia and better understand their sons' behaviors. It's critical to win the trust of this particular group of caregivers, Goff says, to build a multigenerational relationship with Baxter. In families with a genetic predisposition to hemophilia, Baxter has the aspiration to bestow "bleed-free days" for generations to come.

BECOMING A TRUSTED PHARMACIST

Women in our multimarket survey say that trusted pharmacists provide the information customers need to make decisions, ask questions and listen to concerns, discuss options and alternatives, and save customers time. Although this may sound basic, these trust-building behaviors are inconsistently implemented by practitioners. When they are implemented, the gains are enormous.

An example comes from Maria,* an American college student studying abroad in London during the spring of 2013. Within days of moving into her London apartment, Maria was suffering fits of coughing and chronically watering eyes. A double course load and an internship left her pressed for time, so instead of making an appointment at the student health center across town, she went to the corner drugstore. "I was really hoping for a simple solution," she says.

Figure 8.3
WOMEN WHO REPORT THAT THEIR PRIMARY PHARMACIST...
(All markets)

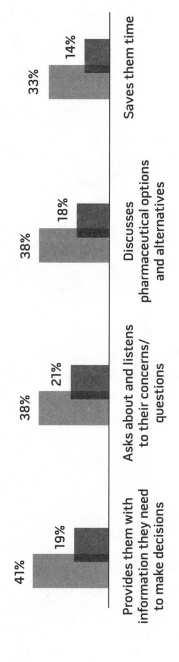

Provides them with information they need to make decisions — 41% / 19%

Asks about and listens to their concerns/questions — 38% / 21%

Discusses pharmaceutical options and alternatives — 38% / 18%

Saves them time — 33% / 14%

Women who are trusting and satisfied with their primary pharmacist
Women who are NOT trusting and satisfied with their primary pharmacist

The pharmacist, seeing her standing perplexed by a wall of identical-looking generic medications, approached her and offered his assistance. He listened patiently as she told her story, interjecting with pertinent questions such as: How long ago did you move here? When did this begin? Has this happened in the past? He concluded that she should try fexofenadine, an antihistamine commonly used to treat symptoms of seasonal allergic rhinitis. He directed her to the generic medication—only £1.50—and told her to please return if her symptoms persisted.

"I couldn't believe how thorough and patient he was," Maria recalls. "It felt just like talking to my doctor back home, except there was no appointment, no inconvenience, and he didn't rush me or condescend to me." He did encourage Maria to purchase a hypoallergenic pillow and, acknowledging that she was new to the city, told her where she could buy one. "I felt like I was talking to someone who really cared and wasn't just trying to sell me something," she explains. "He really was just there to answer my questions and make me better. My symptoms disappeared as soon as I started taking the medicine he recommended."

Walk-in treatment and consultation with pharmacists is common in the UK, where universal healthcare and a cultural acceptance of generic brands keep costs exceedingly low.[37] Pharmacists can offer immediate medical opinions to treat a minor injury or illness or determine that a doctor's visit is necessary. About 85 percent of pharmacies in the UK offer a consultation area where patients and pharmacy staff can discuss issues privately.[38]

With some seventy pharmacies open until midnight nationwide, most of the UK population enjoys access to a pharmacist ready to dispense prescriptions and offer professional advice.[39] Notably, when it comes to medicine, UK patients get over-the-counter medications for pennies on the dollar, and name brands don't compete to sell them medicines that are virtually identical.

The transactional nature of pharmacies in the US tends not to foster trust-building behaviors, explains Kelly Barnes, leader of the US Health Industries Practice at PwC. "For example, in the UK, since healthcare is provided via a nationalized system and you can opt out of that system, there's more opportunity to build brand loyalty with a single pharmacy and pharmacist rather than involving your insurance company to see what medications are covered by your plan," she says. "So convenience and customer relationships matter more."

Intent on building stronger relationships, CVS has created MinuteClinics in more than one hundred of its stores. They're open seven days a week with no appointment necessary, and provide treatments, diagnoses, vaccines, prescriptions, and lab tests for a wide range of common ailments. They also accept most insurance plans.[40] "As the US healthcare system becomes more about out-of-pocket spending and less about insurance coverage of services offered in-network, and we are paying for care directly, the opportunity grows for pharmacists to take on more of the clinical market share," says Barnes.

Walgreens, the largest drug store chain in the US, has also been making moves toward a more customer-centric healthcare experience. New express stations let shoppers skip lines when picking up and paying for their prescriptions. And their long-standing rewards program has recently evolved to reward shoppers for making healthy decisions outside the store, too.

BECOMING A TRUSTED INSURANCE PROVIDER

Complaining about health insurance is common enough in many countries, including the US, but women are clear about what could make them happier: easy, friendly, and informative customer service is what 45 percent of women who trust and are satisfied with their insurance provider say that the company provides. Companies that provide coverage for doctors who women trust, make it easy to find that doctor in-network, and make preventative care affordable also win women's trust across markets.

Take Meredith Ryan-Reid, senior vice president of accident and health worksite benefits at MetLife and time-crunched mother of two. Ryan-Reid noticed that her medical insurance provider had mistakenly sent a claim reimbursement check to her doctor instead of directly to her. So she called the health insurance company, where she encountered menu after menu of options before she could get a customer service

Figure 8.4
WOMEN WHO REPORT THAT THEIR HEALTH INSURANCE COMPANY...
(All markets)

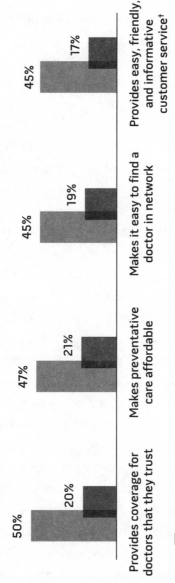

	Provides coverage for doctors that they trust	Makes preventative care affordable	Makes it easy to find a doctor in network	Provides easy, friendly, and informative customer service[†]
Women who are trusting and satisfied	50%	47%	45%	45%
Women who are NOT trusting and satisfied	20%	21%	19%	17%

■ Women who are trusting and satisfied with their health insurance company
■ Women who are NOT trusting and satisfied with their health insurance company

† "Provides easy, friendly, and informative customer service" is a net of "makes it easy to connect to a person when I have a question/claim" and "provides customer service that is friendly and informative"

representative on the line. The service representative then put her on hold. When she finally got back to Ryan-Reid, it was merely to confirm that the company had reimbursed her doctor. "But my insurer made no effort to correct the mistake," says Ryan-Reid. "They wouldn't stop the check, and told me to call my doctor's office, ask that they return my check, and then refile the claim."

Ryan-Reid draws a comparison to her experience with Diapers.com customer service. She remembers making an online order just before a hurricane hit her area. Diapers.com's representative called Ryan-Reid to tell her that the FedEx delivery of her order would be delayed by 24 hours, and that Diapers.com would happily discount her most expensive order by half to compensate for the inconvenience. "They didn't have to do that," she says. "After all, it wasn't their fault that the order was delayed. But, as a result, I will be a customer for life."

Some insurers, thanks to leaders like Ryan-Reid, have undertaken to build trust by listening to what women want. MetLife, for example, has developed a more efficient, more empathetic customer service operation in order to more effectively communicate with employers and their employees. The company strives to be sensitive to time and confidence famines in its service interactions with customers. After all, the majority of MetLife's customers for accident and critical illness coverage are female, and the company's strategy to reach them acts on some of the same insights we uncovered in our survey. "I know if something is easy, given all of the demands on my own time, I'm much more likely to do it," explains Ryan-Reid.

TRANSPARENCY BUILDS TRUST

Another way to increase trust is more transparency. Dr. Leana Wen's online platform Who's My Doctor advocates radical openness; doctors who join the site disclose financial connections to pharmaceutical and medical device companies, reveal their compensation for performing tests and procedures, share personal and professional details, and describe their practice philosophies. This transparent approach seeks to build trust with patients online.

Wen says fear—of malpractice lawsuits, of asking questions, of losing revenue and reputation—has driven patients and doctors away from behaviors that build trust. "When doctors are willing to step off our pedestals, take off our white coats, and show our patients who we are and what medicine is all about—that's when we begin to overcome the sickness of fear. That's when we establish trust," she said in a 2014 TEDMED talk. "That's when we change the paradigm of medicine, from one of secrecy and hiding, to one that is fully open and engaged for our patients."[41]

Wen isn't officially a primary care physician, but as an emergency room doctor, she serves as the sole provider of medical care for many of her emergency room patients. Like Lustig, Wen discovered in her residency that the fast-paced ER culture doesn't welcome doctors who prefer to spend significant time with patients. But instead of opting out, Wen is looking to change the culture. "Some would argue that the ER isn't the right place to deal with people's personal problems," Wen wrote in a recent NPR blog post.[42] "But even now, many of our patients don't see another doctor. These ER visits give us a chance to help them regain their health and also put them on the way toward addressing the underlying issues that affect their well-being."

The same post described several patients who Wen saw in a single day and the women who accompanied them to their appointments. One sixty-seven-year-old man comes in with his wife, who thinks he's having a heart attack. After a long conversation with Wen, it becomes clear that he is trying to stop taking pain medication and is experiencing withdrawal. In her writings, speaking, and advocacy work (besides speaking at TEDMED, she has published a best-selling book entitled *When Doctors Don't Listen*), Wen promotes the clear communication, active listening, and proactive discussions of preventative care that our survey respondents seek. She also tailors her approach for each patient's particular circumstances, better understanding the strain on the patient and their caregiver or decision-maker.[43]

By building a community on the Who's My Doctor platform, Wen is gathering a community of likeminded doctors committed to approaching patients in an inclusive way.

9

Winning in the Marketplace

Winning in the healthcare market place means winning women in their roles as Chief Medical Officers. To meet CMOs' needs and win their trust and loyalty, industry culture has to change, and the change has to start with an inclusive culture that celebrates the power of difference.

Inclusive leadership means managers make it safe for every member on their teams to put bold new ideas on the table. They give actionable feedback and act on the feedback they themselves receive. They empower team members to make decisions and they share credit for team success. And they understand that success requires teams with both "inherent" diversity (e.g. gender, ethnicity, and sexual orientation), as well as the "acquired" diversity derived from different experiences and backgrounds.

It may sound easy, but it's not. Across the board, in healthcare and other sectors, even though women hold over half of all professional-level jobs,[44] they become more and more underrepresented and under-engaged as they climb the ranks. On average, women occupy less than 15 percent of executive positions.[45] The problem is that a company's culture is a rearview mirror: it follows the leadership values, behaviors, decisions, and unconscious biases that were recognized and rewarded in the past. And talent management practices that were constructed, with the best intentions, to be color-blind and gender-blind and treat everyone the same have ended up reinforcing outdated behaviors. Because even as employees, women are different, with unmet needs and distinct customer preferences.

When companies do get it right—when they are gender-smart—the results are impressive.

The research we did at CTI on innovation, diversity, and market growth shows that leadership teams with acquired diversity—whose members have experience living and working abroad, for instance—are more likely to be inclusive.[46] Further research on women in science, engineering, and technology (SET) also reveals that in the pharma and life sciences fields, female leaders are more likely than male leaders to exhibit the behaviors that unlock value and drive innovative outcomes.[47]

Companies that harness the insights of their female talent—whose leaders know how to value the difference that women bring across the entire value chain, from R&D to manufacturing and marketing—are the likeliest to win in the marketplace, as CTI research corroborates. Employees at publicly traded companies with leaders who embody inherent and acquired diversity (which we call 2D Diversity) are 45 percent more likely than

Figure 9.1
EMPLOYEES WHO REPORT THAT THEIR TEAM LEADER...†
(US)

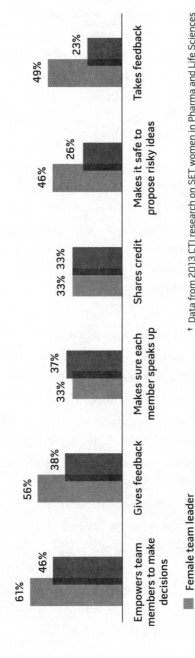

† Data from 2013 CTI research on SET women in Pharma and Life Sciences

employees at publicly traded firms lacking 2D diversity to report that their company has grown its market share in the last year. These employees are also 70 percent more likely to report that their company has captured a new market in the last year.[48]

MISTAKES TO AVOID

The vast majority of large publicly held companies fail to capitalize on their female talent because of a lack of gender smarts at the top: not only are women underrepresented, but too often male leaders have insufficient insight into or appreciation of gender differences. Perhaps because, as our research shows, most employees say that their leaders fail to see value in ideas they personally don't relate to or understand, at companies where senior management is overwhelmingly male, women are less likely than their male colleagues to have their ideas endorsed and implemented. Our findings have been echoed by others: recent research by Google confirms just how important "psychological safety" is for employees to express insights and for teams to function optimally.[49] So it's no surprise that in our study of women in SET fields, we find men at pharmaceutical or life sciences companies to be 24 percent more likely than their female peers to get an idea endorsed.[50]

The psychological toll of working in such an environment can be heavy even for those women who manage to power through to the top. In a recent gathering I facilitated of thirty-five high-potential female leaders in a major pharmaceutical company, along with several men from the company's senior management team, one woman said that after her recent promotion, several male colleagues suggested to her that one of the reasons she got the job was because she was a woman. When I asked the group if anyone else had had a similar experience, every woman raised her hand. The male senior leaders were shocked. Certainly no one had ever insinuated to them that they'd gotten a promotion because they were men.

THE WORK AHEAD

The healthcare industry is an unfortunate example of insufficient diversity at the top: 78 percent of the healthcare workforce is female, but among the forty-five Fortune 500 healthcare companies, not a single one had a woman CEO in 2015 and only about 20 percent of their executives are women.[51] Of the scores of venture-backed digital health start-ups that raised $2 million or more, only three are led by women.[52] Women healthcare professionals are also segmented into lower-status specializations; for example, they comprise only 21 percent of surgeons.[53]

When the leaders all look and think the same, a company's culture is resistant to diverse perspectives—the lifeblood of innovation—and to the talent that can bring these perspectives.

Sophia,* a biotech executive, is an example of how a culture that fails to appreciate diversity can harm a company. Sophia was applauded for her ideas and subject matter expertise, but she soon became alienated when she saw her ideas stalled due to criticism of her communication style. "I got tired of hearing, 'You are the best scientist we have, but you need to change the way you say things: be less direct, less forthcoming,'" Sophia says. "Would they have said that to a man? I doubt it."

Sophia shared her frustration with the CEO and other managers at her company, some of whom attempted to improve the corporate culture's attitudes toward women. But as the company underwent mergers and turnover, inequity in mentorship and leadership opportunities given to women persisted. Sophia continued to feel ignored and ostracized by her direct managers.

Sophia finally left biotech to join an industry publication. She loves her new work environment, which welcomes her ideas and insights. She also started an organization for women in biotech in her area so they can find mentors to support them through the challenges at work.

Women outside the biotech sector tell similar tales. Rachel,* a high-ranking technology leader at a health insurance provider, watched for years as insights shared by women to sell more of the firm's web products to women fell upon deaf ears. To get her own ideas endorsed, Rachel began hiring outside male consultants to deliver them. That way, she told us, her ideas had a far higher likelihood of implementation, even if at a far greater cost to her employer.

Pharmaceutical industry professionals are increasingly aware of the market opportunities their firms may be missing if they're not taking advantage of the insights diversity can bring. "Pharmaceutical companies do enormous amounts of research to better understand how meaningful, differentiated, and innovative therapies can be developed for people living with serious diseases," says Meeta Gulyani, executive vice president and head of Global Strategy and Franchises at Merck Serono. "But we need to explore more than just the biology behind disease."

Companies have a huge strategic opportunity if they learn to communicate better with women as healthcare intermediaries and as colleagues, Gulyani says. "We must go all the way across the healthcare value chain and identify the needs of our customers, particularly women, who are often the decision makers when it comes to health and well-being—for themselves and those around them. We need to better understand the myriad roles women play in shaping the healthcare environment and what their needs are as key contributors to prevention and treatment."

LISTENING TO FEMALE TEAM MEMBERS

In late 2013, Allergan launched Juvederm Voluma XC, the most successful facial filler to hit the market since Botox. It's an FDA-approved gel that can be injected into women's cheeks to correct age-related volume loss and starting from its first year on the market, it's outsold more established players in the cosmetic dermatology arena.

The product's major selling point, according to Michael Jafar, director of marketing at Allergan, is its duration. While the cosmetic effects of competing facial fillers last upward of one year, those of Voluma last two. Voluma's cost is much higher than competing fillers, but for the time-crunched women who buy it, the two-year maintenance schedule more than justifies the expense.

How did Allergan steal away this lucrative market from its household-name-brand competitors? Jafar credits a female member of his team, product manager Cara Chastain, who pushed the team to market the longer-lasting version of Voluma, despite the challenge that its higher price introduced.

Jafar recalls asking his team whether to set a higher price point and push Voluma's long-lasting nature, or to set a lower price point and recommend a three-to-four month touch-up. Along with extensive consumer research, Chastain shared her own perspective. "I'm a parent of two kids," she said. "I will pay a premium not to come back for that touch-up."

Jafar crafted a campaign that stressed the longevity of Voluma's results, and the bet is still paying off. "After extensive market research with our target demographic, and through having conversations with Cara, it became clear to me what was important to our female consumers," Jafar says. "As a result, we gained a significant competitive advantage in the marketplace."

MODELING FEMALE LEADERSHIP

It's one of those ideas that, after it happens, companies wonder why they hadn't done it before: Merck Serono recently placed a woman in charge of its fertility business for the first time.

Dorothea Wenzel has a broad background in healthcare policy from a management consulting career at McKinsey. She also spent ten years in Merck's finance department. Given her diverse healthcare and lived experience, Wenzel is mindful of the patient in her new role. That means that she's brought a new outlook to the company's franchise.

"From the moment I accepted this position, I had women in mind," says Wenzel. "Fifteen years ago, a very close friend of mine opted to try IVF. She told me, 'It's so horrifying for me that I can barely talk about it.'"

Understanding the stigma and stress that accompany fertility treatment has become a major priority for Wenzel. She constantly reminds herself and her team of the struggles and aspirations of the women who use their remedies. "In the pharmaceutical business, we still generally think less about our customers as human beings, but about the physicians as scientific masterminds," Wenzel says. "So we position the product based on the science, and not the human beings who use it. But that's changing." Wenzel began a recent presentation with a photograph of an infant to remind her team of its mission to help women have healthy babies.

Her colleagues responded with an emotional outpouring of praise, saying she was the first leader to so clearly highlight their potential impact. Taking a holistic approach, Wenzel searches for new ways to understand women's stress levels and how they might affect fertility. She also explores ways to make Merck Serono's fertility treatments more affordable through partnerships with financial institutions and clinics. This is especially important for emerging markets and in the United States, where fertility treatments are five to ten times as expensive as they are in Europe.

Wenzel finds the Merck Serono culture open to her new ideas. Another female executive at Merck Serono likewise reported an inclusive culture at the company. Initially employed by Serono, Ada* came to Merck KGaA when the company acquired Serono in a 2006 merger.

"Serono was a bit crazy—we wore bright colors and five-inch heels. They gave women the permission to be authentic. And if you talk to women who were at Merck KGaA corporate headquarters at the time, they were dressing like the men, in black suits, with short hair," Ada says. "Their Serono colleagues gave women the permission to 'come out' as women."

She thinks Merck Serono's female role models encourage women to bring their full selves to the workplace. Ada credits an early sponsor at Serono for her own decision to join the company and bring her ideas to work. But she sees opportunity to better cater to female patients in the development of medicines and devices, especially when it comes to products that are targeted at both men and women. For example, Merck KGaA's fertility injector pen was designed with female professionals in mind, who sought a discrete device that could easily fit in their purses.

But when it comes to the company's multiple sclerosis drug, even though many of the patients are female, those developing the medicine didn't carefully consider the needs of female patients, let alone caregivers or decision makers. Wenzel has her eye on MS as the next opportunity for the company to tap into the power of the purse.

INSIGHTS INTO FEMALE PATIENTS

Pfizer recently created the role of "Global Patient Affairs Lead" for Roslyn Schneider, who worked as a critical care physician and pulmonologist at Beth Israel Medical Center in New York for twenty years. The daughter of immigrants, with seemingly boundless energy, Schneider left Beth Israel to join Pfizer in 2006, rapidly moving through six roles in her eight years with the company to familiarize herself with the business and to find the role that provided the best fit.

She's thrilled to have landed in her current position, where she works to bring in patients' voices at every step of drug development—from the first time patients participate in a human clinical trial to the last time a patient takes one of Pfizer's medicines. And her experience as a woman, she says, continually informs her interactions. "I'm a mom, a wife, and a daughter," she explains. "Those experiences sometimes give me the best gut check." For example, when a colleague told her that they should not assume, in marketing to older women, that women's sexual desire wanes with age, Schneider agreed, explaining that her seventy-nine-year-old mother, far from being shocked by a steamy sex scene at the opening of a film they watched recently, exclaimed, "This looks promising!"

Schneider highly values institutions that have women in senior leadership positions. She notes that Pfizer's female C-suite leaders (including Schneider's supervisor, Chief Medical Officer Freda Lewis-Hall, MD), contribute to her impression of Pfizer as an outstanding employer.

But Pfizer, like all healthcare companies, is still a long way from fully realizing the potential women's insights and a diverse workplace can bring.

In her work heading up global patient affairs, Schneider wants to make existing relationships Pfizer has built with women's advocacy and professional groups more meaningful. "I want to listen even more actively than we have been," she said. She can collaborate with these partners and Pfizer to explore ways to be more inclusive and respond to the information and research they provide.

Schneider's perspective and role at Pfizer demonstrate how companies can explore more inclusive approaches, listen to female insights, and understand where the industry can better meet women's needs and build trust.

WHAT COMPANIES CAN DO

Creating a culture where women feel empowered to share their insights doesn't happen overnight. It takes commitment and consistent messaging across the organization. Leaders have to model inclusivity at every level of management. That said, inclusivity can be taught.

There are tangible steps companies can take to foster a "speak-up culture" that sustains innovation and increases revenue by encouraging and promoting ideas from the talent base that matches their biggest market: women.

1. *Help women win.* Give women the visibility, support, leadership development, and advocacy they need to succeed in the business. The back-office, bench-scientist nature of many health science jobs keeps women off the radar of those

best positioned to help them advance. Building pathways to sponsorship—either by connecting junior women to senior women, or by connecting them to senior men through project or leadership development initiatives—ensures that women get the advocacy and critical feedback they need to assume leadership roles. Junior women aren't likely to "crack the code" of executive presence, let alone break through to leadership, without the input and advocacy of senior men. Just like customers, employees are not monolithic. Companies can benefit by mapping the employee journey to understand employees' needs and experiences as they progress through their lives and careers.

2. *Build an inclusive culture.* Leaders who embrace diversity and behave inclusively create the kind of culture where women come forward with solutions to drive engagement with the female marketplace. Identifying role models of inclusivity is a first step toward codifying, socializing, and rewarding the behaviors that create this "speak-up, listen-down" culture. An inclusive culture knows how to recognize and celebrate the power of difference. Talent management systems—from recruiting, to evaluations, promotions, job assignments and career development—need to become gender-smart. Women may need targeted support in order to fulfill their innovative potential.

3. *Create a differentiated customer experience.* Industry professionals need to recognize that women represent a significant market opportunity because they're decision makers, not just patients and caregivers. Although nearly all women share the same three healthcare famines, to fully engage them as CMOs, companies must recognize how their goals and decision-making factors vary by geography, life situation, and income level. Most importantly, healthcare companies can win women's trust and loyalty as customers by mapping the CMO journey and adopting a holistic definition of health and a partnership approach to serving their needs as patients, caregivers, and consumers.

Figure 9.2
MARKET SUCCESS DEPENDS ON BETTER
UTILIZING FEMALE TALENT

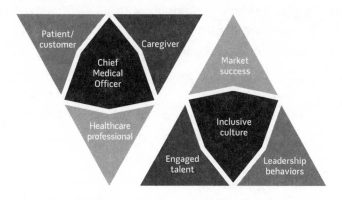

An example of where all of these drivers of success come together is in the deployment of employee resource groups (ERGs). ERGs are traditionally internally focused, representing the needs of their affinity groups. However, progressive healthcare companies are repositioning their charters and recalibrating their aspirations to make ERGs a critical part of solving talent and business-model imperatives for the enterprise. They are, in practice, becoming business resource groups. Leveraging their real-world insights as CMOs, women across all ERGs can spearhead gender-smart initiatives under the sponsorship of inclusive leaders who know how to leverage the power of difference.

HARNESSING THE POWER OF THE PURSE

A focus on women isn't altruism for healthcare companies. It's their best business opportunity.

When companies optimize women's input across the entire value chain, they magnify the likelihood of engaging with key healthcare decision makers—CMOs. Winning women both inside and outside the organization can improve outcomes for their patients and their shareholders.

Eli Lilly is a great case in point. It was the outgoing Chair of the Lilly Women's Network, Eiry Wyn Roberts, MD, VP of Research and Development, and the incoming Chair, Laurie Kowalevsky, Senior Director and Global Brand Leader, Immunology, who led the Lilly sponsorship for the CTI *Power of the Purse* research study. They were convinced that helping Lilly women win inside the company was key to winning in the marketplace and delighting customers.

"Our success in optimizing our desired business outcomes in the marketplace requires that we have exceptional leaders who can fully engage all employees in a way that delivers a positive customer experience for all customers," says Kowalevsky. "Across industries, companies with more female executives have higher returns on equity, higher valuations, better stock performance, and higher payouts of dividends. And it's especially important in healthcare, because women are our main consumers. They're the ones making healthcare decisions. They're the ones we need to understand and reach."

The leadership of the Lilly Women's Network, with the guidance of their executive sponsor, Dave Ricks, recently named CEO, know that gender smarts on the inside and the outside are a business imperative. "Within our own walls at Lilly, we have strong representation of the dominant decision maker and influencer within the space and customers we serve. And we intend to make the most of that," Kowalevsky adds.

Lilly is onto something. By bringing attention to the CMO and segmenting *her* according to her lifestyle, not just the condition of her loved ones, the industry will benefit in many ways. It will...

- boost adherence to prescribed medications, thereby boosting revenue;

- decrease the cost of managing chronic diseases for patients;

- bend the cost curve for claims while improving patients' health outcomes; and

- increase revenue per square foot in pharmacies.

If companies establish a relationship with women that's based on trust, not just transactions, they can also...

- increase returns on R&D investment and

- accelerate their shifts to patient-centered business models.

Women are the drivers behind most healthcare decisions. Companies that learn how to meet their needs will lead—and benefit from—the industry's transformation.

As you'll see in our final chapter, some companies are driving that transformation right now.

10

Taking Action

Since 2015, when we released our *Power of the Purse* study for healthcare, forward-looking healthcare executives and companies have taken action. Some have implemented a gender lens in new parts of the company; others have renewed past efforts or given them a new direction.

All have achieved some success. Many have encountered obstacles. And all agree that there's a lot of work left to do.

In May 2016, I gathered some of the courageous women leaders from the companies that sponsored our research for a "high tea." Assembled around our conference room table, they reflected on their efforts, one year after our study was published.

Here is what we heard.

METLIFE: WOMEN'S INSIGHTS LEAD TO NEW INSURANCE PRODUCTS

When thinking about the development and communication of products, the first questions that Katherine Johnsen Read, director of accident and health product development at MetLife Americas, asks are: Who is the customer I am trying to reach? What are their needs? And how can we build a product to meet those specific needs?

"Understanding who the customer really is—and delivering on their needs—is of utmost importance before beginning any program, initiative, or product," said Johnsen Read.

That's why she was so interested in the findings from our *Power of the Purse* research and Innovation Lab, which showed that the fundamental issue in the healthcare industry is its failure to understand a key customer segment: women.

Given this finding, Johnsen Read thought it would be important to share our research with other women leaders—specifically those who attended MetLife's Annual Women's Global Leadership Forum, part of the Global Women's Initiative that the company started in 2012.

"The research was fascinating," said Johnsen Read. "I knew other women would find it of interest, and I wanted to use the power of our women's group to discuss new ways to reach women."

The result of the forum was outstanding. The participants connected our research with insights already collected from MetLife's customer research to create a fuller picture of the needs, wants, and habits of female insurance customers, particularly in the area of education on supplemental health products.

"Through our customer research, we identified that women are most concerned about out-of-pocket medical and daily expenses that may arise due to an unexpected serious illness or injury, such as an unexpected overnight hospital stay if their child got hurt at a sports game or on the playground," said Johnsen Read. "The *Power of the Purse* research provided additional insight and reinforced our commitment to connecting with women."

MetLife used our research to inform the development of products that were already in the pipeline, including a supplementary health product designed to help women in Europe, the Middle East, and Africa (EMEA) who suffer from certain diseases, such as cervical and breast cancer, reduce their potential out-of-pocket costs.

Johnsen Read is pleased with the work MetLife is doing to address women's needs and knows there's more that can be done.

"We need to constantly be thinking about our customer—who is she, how can we reach her, what are her needs and how are they changing—and develop products and programs accordingly," Johnsen Read said.

Our research showing that women are key healthcare decision-makers also aligned with MetLife's customer insight. "An important part of the information we now provide to our customers and salespeople is that women are the 'Chief Medical Officers'—they're the ones to make healthcare decisions and often make those decisions differently than men."

Looking forward, Johnsen Read is enthusiastic about the possibilities to develop new products and messages that are targeted to women.

"It's powerful to work at a company with both high-profile women leaders and a robust Women's Business Network that takes customer research seriously and acts on it. We're constantly thinking of new ways to reach and help women to meet their personal and family needs."

ELI LILLY AND COMPANY: NEW PROTOCOLS FOR RESEARCH AND DEVELOPMENT

One of the biggest recent developments in the pharmaceutical industry is the move toward customized medicines: the use of genomic information and biomarkers to tailor treatments for specific groups or even specific individuals.

Yet, ever since the modern pharmaceutical industry's start, women have been underrepresented in clinical trials. For many decades, these trials hardly even broke apart the data to see if medications have different impacts on men and women.

Eli Lilly has set about changing that, and though the process had already begun before we published our study, the study's results led the company to "redouble and refocus its efforts," Eiry Wyn Roberts, vice president of Chorus and Exploratory Medicine, says.

"In some cases the genomic information and biomarkers are different across genders. And many of the diseases we're working on are more prevalent among women than among men. So we really had to improve the way our clinical studies worked," she says.

The company has been improving diversity in its clinical trials in race and ethnicity as well as in gender, and it's now applying a gender lens to study the different results. "With a more diverse pool in the clinical trials, we can break down the data. We can look at differences between men and women in terms of how much medication enters the system and how the system responds," Roberts says.

When there is a difference, Lilly then digs in further to see if the difference is just due to body weight, or if— as is sometimes the case—men and women metabolize the medication differently. The company aims to both quantify the degree of variability across gender and find out what's driving the variability.

Lilly is also working to change its entire drug development process to make it more patient-centric. As part of that evolution, it's making women in their role as Chief Medical Officers part of the process for developing clinical studies.

"We've changed our protocols for developing clinical studies," Roberts says. "Before, throughout the pharmaceutical industry, so-called experts, who were overwhelmingly male, designed the studies without consulting much with patients.

"Now, when we plan a clinical study, we include patients and we make an effort to make sure women patients are well-represented. We also include patients' caregivers and decision makers, and we understand that those caregivers and decision-makers are usually women."

The results of this patient-centric approach have been positive, Roberts says: clinical studies that are easier to design and implement. They also have better participation rates, especially among groups like women who were formerly underrepresented.

"You get a lot more buy-in and a lot more participation from patients when they've helped design the study themselves," she says.

CARDINAL HEALTH: GETTING MEN ENGAGED IN CULTIVATING FEMALE TALENT

"Over and over again, the research shows that companies that have more women and cultural diversity in their leadership perform and serve their customers better, attract top talent, have higher employee engagement, and are more innovative," says Carole Watkins, former Chief Human Resources Officer at Cardinal Health. "So we decided that inclusion has to be approached and led with the same attention and importance as any other business imperative. And that means men have to engage actively, too."

Cardinal Health decided to start at the top by naming two men to its two inclusion initiatives: Chairman and CEO George Barrett leads its Diversity and Inclusion Council, and Chief Financial Officer Mike Kaufmann serves as executive sponsor of Cardinal Health's Women's Initiative Network.

"We realized that we'd make more progress if we didn't just have women and ethnically diverse talent talking to each other," Watkins says of the appointments.

She adds that these choices are absolutely not about men "helping" women. "This is about getting men involved in a cultural shift, and building awareness of how unconscious biases and beliefs have the potential to influence behavior and, ultimately, the entire company."

Cardinal Health's program to encourage women in the company had actually begun earlier, with Unconscious Bias training across the organization; with a women's leadership program to help women drive business projects with measurable, significant results; and with setting as a goal diverse slates for all open positions and finding challenging assignments for high potential women and ethnic minorities.

But progress only really began to be significant, Watkins says, after the "Engaging Men for Gender Partnership" initiative began. "That's truly when we began to see our cultural change accelerate," she says.

One prong of the initiative is the Partners Leading Change (PLC) program. PLC features three-day seminars, in which participating men commit to work on a project or initiative that will help transform the company's culture and lead to more women in leadership positions. These projects have included:

- a sponsorship program for women and ethnically diverse talent;

- a program to build support at home for partners of women who work at Cardinal Health; and

- a job rotation program for high-performing women that prepares them for general manager positions.

Nearly 150 male leaders have engaged in the program since its start, says Watkins. "Mike Kaufmann has really been a vocal and committed champion for the program and can be credited with building momentum and excitement around participation," she observes. "Mike's leadership of this program has been an important part of our success."

A second prong of the "Engaging Men for Gender Partnership" initiative is sponsorship. Cardinal Health asked every senior vice president in the organization to sponsor two individuals, one of whom has to be a female and/or ethnically diverse.

"Sponsors advocate for and help build others' recognition of your skills, abilities, and aspirations," Watkins says. "A sponsor is also the one to close the door and give real feedback. Sponsor relationships are not to be entered into lightly. The sponsor has to know the protégé well and be able to see her perform."

Here too, the results have been promising.

"Sponsors are intervening to ensure that the company is retaining, promoting, and recognizing the contributions of their protégés," says Watkins. In addition, the sponsors are learning more from their protégés than imagined, which is an unexpected bonus.

The program has been so successful that some PLC participants developed a project to expand the program to lower levels in the organization. Seventy more leaders, at the VP level, have been trained as sponsors and each selected two protégés, with at least one being female or ethnically diverse.

"All these initiatives together have made a huge difference," Watkins says. "We're not ready to claim victory, but we're more convinced than ever that actively engaging men in our diversity and inclusion initiative is driving the right conversations, awareness, and accountability for this critical business imperative."

"The gender partnership initiative is all about authenticity and engaging men to lean in and learn how to translate diversity and inclusion into their day jobs," said Lisa Gutierrez, vice president of Cardinal Health's Diversity and Inclusion department. "The men didn't wait for the perfect situation, or the perfect context. They just took a step forward and started making a difference in their part of the world, whether with families, colleagues, or their direct reports. The journey is not just about the numbers. It's about embracing the challenges and humbly learning as we go. We are getting clearer on what needles we're trying to move and understanding the outcomes we are trying to achieve."

The initiative has already helped lead to tangible results. The company's inclusion index, which is part of the annual "Voice of the Employee" survey, has increased year over year with single digit percentage points. Overall turnover between men and women at the manager level is at a comparable rate.

"The business case for sponsorship, not just of women, but of ethnic minorities too, has been proven," Watkins says. "We've made progress, but we still have work to do."

GHG | GREYHEALTH GROUP: SEIZING A MARKETING AND COMMUNICATIONS OPPORTUNITY

To serve the $6.5 trillion healthcare market, industry players are developing amazing products, healthcare is more widely available than ever before, and technology has brought an explosion of health information directly to patients and consumers. Yet patients and consumers continue to falter when it comes to caring for their own health.

In order to find the source of the problem, ghg | greyhealth group commissioned research to build on the CTI study and determine whether healthcare professionals are aware of how they are perceived by the women who are making the healthcare decisions, termed Chief Health Officers (CHO) by ghg. The study was designed to measure the depth of the disconnect between women and their healthcare partners and to point toward new ways to speak with women that involve moving beyond direct ad campaigns to a far more extensive dialogue.

The survey revealed a startling gulf between the types of communication that CHOs claim they need to care for their families' health and what primary care providers, pharmacists, and managed care organizations believe they actually offer. In every case, the healthcare professionals gave themselves far higher scores than their female patients gave them. The study not only confirmed that there is a huge disconnect between the percentage of healthcare providers who say that their female customers trust them, and the percentage of women who actually do trust them, but that healthcare providers are largely unaware of their own failings.

These revealing findings offer those in marketing communications a golden opportunity to develop more meaningful messaging and tools and prove further that communication is the way to properly prepare women to be effective, even revolutionary, healthcare advocates. Because right now, although women make the majority of healthcare decisions, they don't have the tools or the trusted partners to make good ones.

The behaviors that build trust and confidence aren't complex. Women want to save time, receive clear information, and have their concerns heard.

"What women really want is communication," says ghg CEO Lynn O'Connor Vos. "They want communication that is more honest, more understandable, more immediate, and more actionable."

With our report and its own further research in hand, ghg has prepared several new marketing campaigns and won new clients based on their understanding of women's role in healthcare decision making.

"It is important in today's environment to create a conversation, and ideally one that is fully transparent," says O'Connor Vos. "Women appreciate marketers that share all of the facts and provide information and resources to help them make educated decisions."

She says that ghg's evident expertise on the CHO has given the firm itself ways to stand out from the crowd of communications companies. It's become a very big part of their client presentations.

"This research has given us a tremendous opportunity for partnership, publicity, and leadership. We've had many clients invite us to speak about it," says O'Connor Vos.

The media has also paid attention. Since the firm published its white paper on women as chief health officers in November 2015, and increased its emphasis on women as healthcare decision makers, *Fortune Magazine*, *PRWeek*, and *AdWeek* have all devoted feature articles to ghg's ideas and campaigns aimed at women.

Finally, the focus on women has proven perfectly aligned with ghg's other main emphasis: on communicating with that other holy grail of marketing targets, the generation of millennials.

"When you look at what women want and at what millennials want, there's a lot of overlap," O'Connor Vos says. "They both define health to include mental and emotional well-being, with an emphasis on lowering stress. They both want not to be passive consumers, but to have more interaction with their healthcare providers. They want information.

"As millennials become the dominant consumer group, many of the same strategies that apply to women will apply to them, too," she adds. "It all boils down to ghg's mantra: communication is the cure. And women and millennials are listening."

JOHNSON & JOHNSON: REACHING OUTSIDE THE CORPORATE WORLD FOR PARTNERS

Johnson & Johnson has long recognized that diversity in senior leadership positions is a business imperative. "We fully believe that having a diverse group of executives at the table, making critical decisions and driving our strategy, provides new perspectives, increases creativity, and helps lead to the innovation that will grow the company," says Wanda Bryant Hope, chief diversity officer for Johnson & Johnson. Bringing more women into senior ranks is particularly important because of women's role as healthcare decision makers, Hope adds.

"By facilitating female leaders' rise into higher-level roles in our organization, we increase our capabilities to design, develop, and market products to women in their roles as 'Chief Medical Officers' with their families in mind."

In order to meet this need, for the last fourteen years, J&J has collaborated with Smith College, a renowned women-only higher education institution in the US. Together, J&J executives and Smith College professors designed a training program tailored to the needs of high-potential women at J&J, to increase retention rates and help them realize their potential to contribute to the company.

The Smith Custom Leadership Development Program is one week of intensive classwork, capability building, networking opportunities, peer coaching, and interactive exercises, including an all-day business simulation that gives participants the experience of running the company. The program's teaching staff includes both Smith College professors and J&J executives at the vice president level and higher. The participants are women in entry-level management positions.

Lots of research, including some conducted by CTI, has found that talented women drop out more and more at each step up the management ladder. The idea behind J&J's Smith Custom program is to ensure that women have the skills, advice, coaching, and support needed to continue their success.

"The program is focused on further accelerating female talent through our pipeline. It gives high-potential women the skills they need to navigate the organizational ladder, early in their careers," says Elvie Gee, program management officer of diversity and talent management at Johnson & Johnson, who oversees the program.

The program began by bringing sixty women a year, with representation from every region of J&J's global operations, to the company's headquarters in New Jersey. In light of its success, J&J in 2011 began offering the program twice a year, so 120 women now participate annually in the US. Since demand from abroad has been so strong, J&J last year expanded the program to the Asia Pacific region, bringing those women leaders to one of the company's hubs in Singapore.

"We've always brought high potential women in from Asia, as we do from every other region, to participate in the program in the US, and we're still doing that," Gee says. "But we realized we could reach a lot more women in a key region if we also offered the program in Asia."

Just as in the US, the Singapore program is a collaboration between J&J executives and Smith College faculty, but it also includes university professors from Singapore to ensure local and regional relevance. "It was important for us to adapt the program and content for local needs. We knew that simply transplanting the US program with no changes would be far less effective," Gee says. With the Asia program also a success, Gee says J&J is currently evaluating offering similar programs, customized for local needs, to entry-level female executives in other parts of the world.

IN CLOSING

A Personal Note

I've been working in the private sector for over forty years. That period coincides almost exactly with the various phases of the modern Women's Movement. One success of that movement is that today, getting more women into senior ranks in the private and public sectors is a priority. But for all the various strategies, plans, and announcements of good intentions, business leaders remain skeptical that bringing more women into leadership will measurably improve the bottom line. They ask, or would like to ask, "Why are we bothering? What's the business purpose here?" Or they'll say, "Give me something concrete to motivate change!"

Answering this lingering question has become the center of my professional life. It's the reason why I go to work each day with even more passion and enthusiasm than when I was fresh out of college. The business case for getting more women into the executive ranks of healthcare companies is this: *without them, companies won't be able to save lives, bring down costs, or retain market share, let alone grow it.*

Women have long been recognized for the unique role they play in families, communities, and society. They shepherd us into the world and mourn us as we take leave of it. They work daily to keep us safe and well-cared for, supporting us in sickness and in health. It's time their roles as CMOs and as committed healthcare professionals also be acknowledged. Because if we listen to women, if we celebrate their insights and efforts, allow them to fully claim their ambition, and give them a place at the table, then we'll hit the trifecta: individuals, societies, and companies all benefit.

Now that's something we can all get passionate about.

ENDNOTES

1. "Number, Rate, and Average Length of Stay for Discharges from Short-Stay Hospitals, by Age, Region, and Sex: United States, 2010," Centers for Disease Control and Prevention, 2010, http://www.cdc.gov/nchs/data/nhds/1general/2010gen1 _agesexalos.pdf; "General Facts on Women and Job Based Health," United States Department of Labor, December 2013, http://www.dol.gov/ebsa/newsroom/fshlth5.html; "Women and Health Care: A National Profile," Kaiser Family Foundation, July 2005, https://kaiserfamilyfoundation.files.wordpress .com/2013/01/women-and-health-care-a-national-profile-key -findings-from-the-kaiser-women-s-health-survey.pdf.

2. Catalyst, "Women in Medicine," Catalyst Inc., 2012, http://www.catalyst.org/knowledge/women-medicine; "Executive Summary: Caregiving in the US," National Alliance for Caregiving in collaboration with AARP, 2009, http://www .caregiving.org/pdf/research/CaregivingUSAllAgesExecSum.pdf.

3. Catalyst, *Buying Power: Global Women* (New York: Catalyst, 2015), http://www.catalyst.org/knowledge/buying-power -global-women.

4. "Fast Facts: Marketing to Women," PME Enterprises LLC, accessed August 3, 2016, http://m2w.biz/fast-facts/.

5. Capgemini Consulting, "Patient Adherence: The Next Frontier in Patient Care," Capgemini, 2011, http://www.pt.capgemini.com /resource-file-access/resource/pdf/Patient_Adherence__The _Next_Frontier_in_Patient_Care.pdf.

6. Ernst & Young, *Progressions: The Third Place: Healthcare Everywhere* (Boston: Global Life Sciences Center, 2012).

7. Sundiantu Dixon-Fyle, Shonu Gandhi, and Angela Spatharou, "Changing Patient Behavior: The Next Frontier in Healthcare Value," Health International, McKinsey & Company, 2012, http://healthcare.mckinsey.com/changing-patient-behavior -next-frontier-healthcare-value.

8. Matthias Evers et al., "Pharma Medical Affairs: 2020 and Beyond," McKinsey & Company, July 2014, http://www .mckinsey.com/insights/health_systems_and_services/pharma _medical_affairs_2020_and_beyond.

9. Basel Kayyali, David Knott, and Steve Van Kulken, "The Big-Data Revolution in US Health Care: Accelerating Value and Innovation," McKinsey & Company, April 2013, http://www.mckinsey.com/insights/health_systems _and_services/the_big -data_revolution_in_us_health_care.

10. Jonathan Anscombe et al., "Building Value-Based Healthcare Business Models," Pharma in Europe: New Medicine for a New World, A.T. Kearney, 2013, http://www.atkearney.com /documents/10192/2719243/Building +Value-Based +Healthcare+Business+Models.pdf/6b3065e1-a1e3-4e82-8477 -0903bcdc68af.

11. Beena Jimmy and Jimmy Jose, "Patient Medication Adherence: Measures in Daily Practice," *Oman Medical Journal* 26, no. 3 (May 2011): 155-159, doi:10.5001/omj.2011.38.

12. "Hemant Ahlawat, Giulia Chierchia, and Paul van Arkel, "The Secret of Successful Drug Launches," McKinsey & Company, March 2014, http://www.mckinsey.com/industries/pharma ceuticals-and-medical-products/our-insight/the-secret-of -successful-drug-launches.

13. "Total Global Pharmaceutical Spending on Research and Development from 2006 to 2020 (in Billion US Dollars)," Statista, 2016, http://www.statista.com/statistics/309466/global-r-and -d-expenditure-for-pharmaceuticals/.

14. Cristina Boccuti and Giselle Casillas, "Aiming for Fewer Hospital U-turns: The Medicare Hospital Readmision Reduction Program," Kaiser Family Foundation, January 29, 2015, http://kff.org/medicare/issue-brief/aiming-for-fewer-hospital-u -turns-the-medicare-hospital-readmission-reduction-program/.

15. Jason M. Thomas and Stephen H. Wise, 2016 Global Health Care Outlook (Washington, DC: The Carlyle Group, November 2015), https://www.carlyle.com/sites/default/files/market -commentary/october_2015_-_global_health_care_investment _outlook.pdf; "Medical Cost Trend: Behind the Numbers 2017," PwC, accessed August 1, 2016, http://www.pwc.com /us/en/health-industries/health-research-institute/behind-the -numbers.html.

16. "Jobs to Be Done," Clayton Christensen Institute for Disruptive Innovation, accessed August 1, 2016, http://www .christenseninstitute.org/key-concepts/jobs-to-be-done/.

17. Catalyst, "Women in Medicine" (see note 2).

18. Sylvia Ann Hewlett, Melinda Marshall, and Laura Sherbin, with Tara Gonsalves, *Innovation, Diversity and Market Growth* (New York: Center for Talent Innovation, 2013), 5.

19. Ibid, 51.

20. Zach Gerber and Kit Shea, *Millennial Mindset: The Worried Well* (New York: Allidura, 2014), http://allidura.com/downloads/141020_millennial_report.pdf.

21. "Magnolia Meals at Home," Eisai Incorporated, 2015, http://www.magnoliamealsathome.com/-/media/Files/MagnoliaMealsAtHome/final-program-brochure.pdf?la=en.

22. "Chronic Diseases and Health Promotion," World Health Organization, accessed February 18, 2015, http://www.who.int/chp/en/.

23. "OECD Family Database," OECD, 2014, http://www.oecd.org/social/family/database.htm.

24. Katrin Bennhold, "The Good Mother and Modern Politician," *New York Times*, January 17, 2010, http://www.nytimes.com/2010/01/18/world/europe/18iht-womenside.html.

25. Ibid.

26. Ursula von der Leyen, interview by Flora Wisdorff, "Mir geht es besser, wenn ich Tiere um michhabe," Die Welt, April 4, 2013, http://www.welt.de/wirtschaft/article118662554/Mir-geht-es-besser-wenn-ich-Tiere-um-mich-habe.html.

27. "Amanda Hinchcliffe: Life as a Sandwich Carer," Carers UK, accessed July 27, 2016, http://www.carersuk.org/help-and-advice/health/looking-after-your-health/caring-for-your-back/2839:life-as-a-sandwich-carer.

28. "Facts," Anxiety and Depression Association of America, accessed August 1, 2016, http://www.adaa.org/living-with-anxiety/women/facts.

29. Jodi Kantor, "Working Anything but 9 to 5," *New York Times*, August 13, 2014, http://www.nytimes.com/interactive/2014/08/13/us/starbucks-workers-scheduling-hours.html.

30. Eric J. Topol, "The Future of Medicine Is in Your Smartphone," *Wall Street Journal*, January 9, 2015, http://www.wsj.com/articles/the-future-of-medicine-is-in-your-smartphone-1420828632.

31. Michella Llamas, "How the FDA Let Women Down," Drug Watch, accessed August 3, 2016, https://www.drugwatch.com /fda-let-women-down/.

32. Janine Austin Clayton, "Filling the Gaps: NIH to Enact New Policies to Address Sex Differences,"National Institute of Health: Office of Research on Women's Health, May 14, 2014, http://orwh.od.nih.gov/about/director/director_nature_2014.asp.

33. "Cooper, Lummis Reintroduce Research for All Act," United States Congressman Jim Cooper, May 5, 2015, https://cooper .house.gov/media-center/press-releases/cooper-lummis -reintroduce-research-for-all-act.

34. 114th Congress, "H.R.2101 – Research for All Act of 2015," Congress.gov, accessed August 30, 2016, https://www.congress .gov/bill/114th-congress/house-bill/2101.

35. Phil Wahba, "The Change Agent inside CVS," *Fortune*, September 11, 2015, http://fortune.com/2015/09/11/cvs -health-helena-foulkes/.

36. "CVS Health," *Fortune*, accessed July 28, 2016, http://fortune .com/worlds-most-admired-companies/cvs-health-27/.

37. Kim Gittleson, "Walgreens to Buy Up Alliance Boots," BBC, August 6, 2014, http://www.bbc.com/news/business-28674140.

38. "Pharmacy Services," NHS Choices, 2014, http://www.nhs .uk/NHSEngland/AboutNHSservices/pharmacists/Pages /pharmacistsandchemists.aspx.

39. "Late Night Pharmacy," The Boots Company PLC, accessed August 1, 2016, http://www.boots.com/en/Pharmacy-Health /Health-information/Midnight-Pharmacy/.

40. "Services," CVS Minute Clinic, 2014, http://www.cvs.com /minuteclinic/services.

41. Leana Wen, "What Your Doctors Won't Disclose," TED video, 15:42, posted September 2014, http://www.ted.com/talks /leana_wen_what_your_doctor_won_t_disclose?language=en.

42. Leana Wen, "Why the ER Doctor Asks Patients What's Happening at Home," National Public Radio, November 29, 2014, http://www.npr.org/blogs/health/2014/11/20 /365503118/why-the-er-doctor-asks-patients-whats -happening-at-home.

43. Leana Wen and Joshua Kosowsky, *When Doctors Don't Listen: How to Avoid Misdiagnoses and Unnecessary Tests* (New York: St. Martin's Press, 2012).

44. Judith Warner, "Fact Sheet: The Women's Leadership Gap," Center for American Progress, March 7, 2014, https://www .americanprogress.org/issues/women/report/2014/03/07 /85457/fact-sheet-the-womens-leadership-gap/.

45. Ibid.

46. Hewlett et al., *Innovation* (see note 18).

47. Unpublished data from Sylvia Ann Hewlett and Laura Sherbin, with Fabiola Dieudonné, Christina Fargnoli, and Catherine Fredman, *Athena Factor 2.0: Accelerating Female Talent in Science, Engineering & Technology* (New York: Center for Talent Innovation, 2014); see also: Carolyn Buck Luce, Sylvia Ann Hewlett, Julia Taylor Kennedy, and Laura Sherbin, *The Power of the Purse: Engaging Women Decision Makers for Healthy Outcomes* (New York: Center for Talent Innovation 2015).

48. Hewlett et al., *Innovation* (see note 18).

49. Charles Duhigg, "What Google Learned from Its Quest to Build the Perfect Team," *New York Times*, February 25, 2016, http://www.nytimes.com/2016/02/28/magazine/what-google -learned-from-its-quest-to-build-the-perfect-team.html?_r=2.

50. Unpublished data from Hewlett, et al., *Athena Factor* (see note 47).

51. Diljot Chhina, "The State of Healthcare Gender Diversity 2016," Rock Health, January 18, 2016, https://rockhealth.com/the -state-of-healthcare-gender-diversity-2016/.

52. Rock Health, "Women in Healthcare," Rock Health, January 5, 2012, http://www.slideshare.net/RockHealth/rock-report -iii-women-in-healthcare?qid=ef32aed2-4192-4a62-a9af -09e53e191953&v=default&b=&from_search=2.

53. American College of Surgeons and Health Policy Research Institute, "The Surgical Workforce in the United States: Profile and Recent Trends," Association of American Medical Colleges, 2010, http://www.acshpri.or/documents/ACSHPRI_Surgical _Workforce_in_US_apr2010.pdf.

APPENDIX:
HEALTH LITERACY QUIZ

1. Which of these food classifications DOES NOT provide the body with energy?

- ☐ Calories
- ☐ Protein
- ☐ Vitamins
- ☐ Carbohydrates
- ☐ Fat

2. Which organ in the body produces insulin?

- ☐ Liver
- ☐ Small Intestines
- ☐ Stomach
- ☐ Kidneys
- ☐ Pancreas

3. The disease where abnormal cells divide uncontrollably in a part of the body and can invade other tissues is called...

- ☐ Hypertension
- ☐ Malaria
- ☐ Tuberculosis
- ☐ Cancer
- ☐ HIV/AIDS

4. Which of these is/are a sexually transmitted disease? *Select all that apply:*

☐ Leukemia

☐ Crohn's Disease

☐ Syphilis

☐ Gonorrhea

☐ Chlamydia

5. Please match up the following words with their definitions:

_ Anemia
    a. The time in a woman's life when menstruation stops

_ Jaundice
    b. Medicine that fights bacterial infections

_ Menopause
    c. Causes the yellowing of the skin and whites of the eyes

_ Antibiotic
    d. A condition in which the body does not have enough healthy red blood cells, which can result in feeling exhausted

6. Bad breath that persists and gums that bleed easily are symptoms of...

☐ Periodontal disease

☐ Irritable bowel syndrome

☐ High blood pressure

☐ Heart disease

☐ Osteoporosis

7. What causes the common cold?

- ☐ Diabetes
- ☐ Mold and fungi
- ☐ Virus
- ☐ An allergic reaction
- ☐ Bacteria

8. Which of the following are health effects of smoking cigarettes? *Select all that apply:*

- ☐ Stroke
- ☐ Lung cancer
- ☐ Chronic obstructive pulmonary disease (COPD)
- ☐ Hepatitis C
- ☐ There are no health effects to smoking cigarettes

Answers:
1. Vitamins; 2. Pancreas; 3. Cancer; 4. Syphilis, Gonorrhea, Chlamydia; 5a. Menopause; 5b. Antibiotic; 5c. Jaundice; 5d. Anemia; 6. Periodontal disease; 7. Virus; 8. Stroke, Lung cancer, Chronic obstructive pulmonary disease (COPD).

METHODOLOGY OF THE CTI STUDY

The CTI research cited in this book consists of a survey, Insights In-Depth° sessions (a proprietary web-based tool used to conduct voice-facilitated virtual focus groups) involving more than 120 people from our Task Force organizations, and one-on-one interviews with 72 men and women in the US, UK, Germany, Japan, and Brazil.

The survey was conducted by Kantar Health under the auspices of the Center for Talent Innovation, a nonprofit research organization. Kantar Health was responsible for the data collection, while the Center for Talent Innovation conducted the analysis.

The Center for Talent Innovation collaborated with Kantar Health to prepare a custom follow-up online survey to the National Health and Wellness Survey (NHWS). The NHWS is the largest healthcare database of projectable, self-reported, real-world patient-level information. Prior inclusion in NHWS was required to link results across the two studies.

The custom survey was conducted online in July 2014 through September 2014 among 9,218 respondents (4,546 men and 4,672 women: 2,040 in the US,

2,095 in the UK, 2,097 in Germany, 2,089 in Japan, and 897 in Brazil) ages eighteen and up. The NHWS results were from 2013 in the US, UK, Germany, and Japan and 2012 in Brazil. Data from NHWS and custom survey were weighted on gender and age in all geographies. The base used for statistical testing was the effective base.

In the charts, percentages may not always add up to 100 because of computer rounding or the acceptance of multiple responses from respondents.

ACKNOWLEDGMENTS

I am deeply grateful to the study sponsors—Aetna, Bristol-Myers Squibb, Cardinal Health, Eli Lilly and Company, Johnson & Johnson, Merck & Co., Merck KGaA, MetLife, Pfizer, PwC, Strategy&, Teva, and WPP—for their generous support.

Thanks especially to those who participated in interviews—Teri Aronowitz, Rita Balice-Gordon, Kelly Barnes, David Berman, Celia Besore, Lyla Blake-Gumbs, Natalie Bowersox, Margery Brittain, Reid Carpenter, Amy Compton-Phillips, Lisa Courtade, Michelle Cuccia, Jorge Daboub, Ysabel Duron, Elcin Ergun, Miriam Faid, Sandra Fenwick, Simone Fishburn, Susan Fox, Susan Franks, Amy Fry, Venus Ginés, Brian Goff, Ellen Gold, John Gray, Meeta Gulyani, Dawn Halkuff, Patti Harvey, Sharonne Hayes, Bridgette Heller, Sue Herbert, Shanna Hoffman, Sandra Humbles, Mike Jafar, Phyllis Jarrett-Sutton, Minoo Javanmardian, Shireen Jayne, Annalisa Jenkins, Anne Klibanski, Felicitas Lacbawan, DJ Larson, Risa Lavizzo-Mourey, Daniel Lawlor, Lili Lustig, Barbara McGuire, Margaret McKenzie, Alexa Meara, Susan Medansky, Christina Meringolo, Virginia Miller, Sean Morrison, Dan Movens, Niven Narain, Ryoji Noritake, Susan Othello, Gary Pelletier, Brenda Raphael, Katherine Read, Regine Remy, Rochelle Rosian, Meredith Ryan-

Reid, Eric Salama, Gudrun Schmidt, Roslyn Schneider, Karen Scollick, Anjali Shah, Keiko Sheriff, Dawn Sherman, Elke Simon, Sirilak Suteekul, Monica Svets, Jo Taylor, Jeanne Varrone, Lauren Weintraub, Dorothea Wenzel, Axel Wiest—and all the women and men who took part in focus groups, Insights In-Depth® sessions, and all other qualitative research.

We deeply appreciate the efforts of the CTI team, specifically Noni Allwood, Justin Bilyeu, Diana Forster, Kennedy Ihezie, and Peggy Shiller. Thanks also to Roxanna Azari, Danielle Cruz, Colin Elliott, Jessica Jia, Becky Midura, Ripa Rashid, Brandon Urquhart, and Eunice Yu for their support. We also wish to thank Kathy Annunziata, Mike Kelly, Sheila Mott, Eugenia Peck, Julia Zhang, and the team at Kantar Health who expertly guided the research and were an invaluable resource throughout the course of this study.

Thanks also to the cochairs of the Task Force for Talent Innovation—Redia Anderson, Cynthia Bowman, Erika Irish Brown, Deb Bubb, Yrthya Dinzey-Flores, Deborah Elam, Gail Fierstein, Cassandra Frangos, Trevor Gandy, David Gonzales, Wanda Hope, Rosalind Hudnell, Renee Johnson, Patricia Langer, Kate Nekic-Padgett, Kendall O'Brien, Lisa Garcia Quiroz, Craig Robinson, Shari Slate, David Tamburelli, Eileen Taylor, Nancy Testa, Karyn Twaronite, Anré Williams, and Melinda Wolfe—for their vision and commitment, and to the other private sector members of the Task Force for Talent Innovation for their practical ideas and collaborative energy.

ADDITIONAL PUBLICATIONS

KEEPING TALENTED WOMEN ON THE ROAD TO SUCCESS

Ambition in Black and White: The Feminist Narrative Revised
Center for Talent Innovation, June 2016

The Power of the Purse: Engaging Women Decision Makers for Healthy Outcomes
Sponsors: Aetna, Bristol-Myers Squibb, Cardinal Health, Eli Lilly and Company, Johnson & Johnson, Merck & Co., Merck KGaA, MetLife, Pfizer, PwC, Strategy&, Teva, WPP (2015)

Women Want Five Things
Sponsors: American Express, AT&T, Bank of America, Boehringer Ingelheim USA, Merck KGaA, The Moody's Foundation (2014)

Harnessing the Power of the Purse: Female Investors and Global Opportunities for Growth
Sponsors: Credit Suisse, Deutsche Bank, Goldman Sachs, Morgan Stanley, Standard Chartered Bank, UBS (2014)

Executive Presence: The Missing Link between Merit and Success
HarperCollins, June 2014

Forget a Mentor, Find a Sponsor: The New Way to Fast-Track Your Career
Harvard Business Review Press, September 2013

On-Ramps and Up-Ramps India
Sponsors: Citi, Genpact, Sodexo, Standard Chartered Bank,
Unilever (2013)

Executive Presence
Sponsors: American Express, Bloomberg LP, Credit Suisse,
Ernst & Young, Gap Inc., Goldman Sachs, Interpublic Group,
The Moody's Foundation (2012)

Sponsor Effect 2.0: Road Maps for Sponsors and Protégés
Sponsors: American Express, AT&T, Booz Allen Hamilton,
Deloitte, Freddie Mac, Genentech, Morgan Stanley (2012)

Sponsor Effect: UK
Sponsor: Lloyds Banking Group (2012)

**Off-Ramps and On-Ramps Japan: Keeping Talented Women
on the Road to Success**
Sponsors: Bank of America, Cisco, Goldman Sachs (2011)

The Relationship You Need to Get Right
Harvard Business Review, October 2011

Sponsor Effect: Breaking Through the Last Glass Ceiling
Sponsors: American Express, Deloitte, Intel, Morgan Stanley
(2010)

Off-Ramps and On-Ramps Revisited
Harvard Business Review, June 2010

Off-Ramps and On-Ramps Revisited
Sponsors: Cisco, Ernst & Young, The Moody's Foundation
(2010)

Letzte Ausfahrt Babypause
Harvard Business Manager (Germany), May 2010

Off-Ramps and On-Ramps Germany
Sponsors: Boehringer Ingelheim, Deutsche Bank, Siemens AG
(2010)

*Off-Ramps and On-Ramps: Keeping Talented Women on the
Road to Success*
Harvard Business Review Press, 2007

*Off-Ramps and On-Ramps: Keeping Talented Women on the
Road to Success*
Harvard Business Review, March 2005

*The Hidden Brain Drain: Off-Ramps and On-Ramps in
Women's Careers*
Sponsors: Ernst & Young, Goldman Sachs, Lehman Brothers
(2005)

LEVERAGING MINORITY AND MULTICULTURAL TALENT

Black Women: Ready to Lead
Sponsors: American Express, AT&T, Bank of America, Chubb
Group of Insurance Companies, The Depository Trust &
Clearing Corporation, Intel, Morgan Stanley, White & Case
LLP (2015)

*How Diversity Drives Innovation: A Compendium of Best
Practices*
Sponsors: Bloomberg LP, Bristol-Myers Squibb, Cisco,
Deutsche Bank, EY, Siemens AG, Time Warner (2014)

*Cracking the Code: Executive Presence and Multicultural
Professionals*
Sponsors: Bank of America, Chubb Group of Insurance
Companies, Deloitte, GE, Intel Corporation, McKesson
Corporation (2013)

How Diversity Can Drive Innovation
Harvard Business Review, December 2013

Innovation, Diversity and Market Growth
Sponsors: Bloomberg LP, Bristol-Myers Squibb, Cisco,
Deutsche Bank, EY, Siemens AG, Time Warner (2013)

**Vaulting the Color Bar: How Sponsorship Levers
Multicultural Professionals into Leadership**
Sponsors: American Express, Bank of America, Bristol-Myers
Squibb, Deloitte, Intel, Morgan Stanley, NBCUniversal (2012)

**Asians in America: Unleashing the Potential of the "Model
Minority"**
Sponsors: Deloitte, Goldman Sachs, Pfizer, Time Warner (2011)

**Sin Fronteras: Celebrating and Capitalizing on the Strengths
of Latina Executives**
Sponsors: Booz Allen Hamilton, Cisco, Credit Suisse, General
Electric, Goldman Sachs, Johnson & Johnson, Time Warner
(2007)

Global Multicultural Executives and the Talent Pipeline
Sponsors: Citigroup, General Electric, PepsiCo, Time Warner,
Unilever (2008)

**Leadership in Your Midst: Tapping the Hidden Strengths of
Minority Executives**
Harvard Business Review, November 2005

**Invisible Lives: Celebrating and Leveraging Diversity in the
Executive Suite**
Sponsors: General Electric, Time Warner, Unilever (2005)

**Forthcoming 2016: *Latinos at Work: Unleashing the Power of
Culture***

REALIZING THE FULL POTENTIAL OF LGBT TALENT

Out in the World: Securing LGBT Rights in the Global Marketplace
Sponsors: American Express, Bank of America, Barclays, Bloomberg LP, BNY Mellon, BP, Chubb Group of Insurance Companies, Deutsche Bank, Eli Lilly and Company, Ernst & Young LLP, and Out Leadership (2016)

The Power of "Out" 2.0: LGBT in the Workplace
Sponsors: Deloitte, Out on the Street, Time Warner (2013)

For LGBT Workers, Being "Out" Brings Advantages
Harvard Business Review, July/August 2011

The Power of "Out": LGBT in the Workplace
Sponsors: American Express, Boehringer Ingelheim USA, Cisco, Credit Suisse, Deloitte, Google (2011)

RETAINING AND SUSTAINING TOP TALENT

Mission Critical: Unlocking the Value of Vets in the Workforce
Sponsors: Booz Allen Hamilton, Boehringer Ingelheim USA, Fordham University, Intercontinental Exchange/NYSE, Prudential Financial, The Moody's Foundation, Wounded Warrior Project (2015)

Top Talent: Keeping Performance Up When Business Is Down
Harvard Business Press, 2009

Sustaining High Performance in Difficult Times
Sponsor: The Moody's Foundation (2008)

Seduction and Risk: The Emergence of Extreme Jobs
Sponsors: American Express, BP plc, ProLogis, UBS (2007)

Extreme Jobs: The Dangerous Allure of the 70-Hour Workweek
Harvard Business Review, December 2006

Forthcoming 2017: *Disrupting Bias, Uncovering Value*

TAPPING INTO THE STRENGTHS OF GEN Y, GEN X, AND BOOMERS

Misunderstood Millennial Talent: The Other Ninety-One Percent
Sponsors: American Express, Baxalta, Ernst & Young LLP, The Moody's Foundation, Novo Nordisk, S&P Global (2016)

The X Factor: Tapping into the Strengths of the 33- to 46-Year-Old Generation
Sponsors: American Express, Boehringer Ingelheim USA, Cisco, Credit Suisse, Google (2011)

How Gen Y & Boomers Will Reshape Your Agenda
Harvard Business Review, July/August 2009

Bookend Generations: Leveraging Talent and Finding Common Ground
Sponsors: Booz Allen Hamilton, Ernst & Young, Lehman Brothers, Time Warner, UBS (2009)

BECOMING A TALENT MAGNET IN EMERGING MARKETS

Growing Global Executives: The New Competencies
Sponsors: American Express, Bloomberg LP, Cisco Systems, EY, Genpact, Goldman Sachs, Intel, Pearson, Sodexo, The Moody's Foundation (2015)

The Battle for Female Talent in Brazil
Sponsors: Bloomberg LP, Booz & Company, Intel, Pfizer,
Siemens AG (2011)

Winning the War for Talent in Emerging Markets
Harvard Business Press, August 2011

The Battle for Female Talent in China
Sponsors: Bloomberg LP, Booz & Company, Intel, Pfizer,
Siemens AG (2010)

The Battle for Female Talent in India
Sponsors: Bloomberg LP, Booz & Company, Intel, Pfizer,
Siemens AG (2010)

The Battle for Female Talent in Emerging Markets
Harvard Business Review, May 2010

PREVENTING THE EXODUS OF WOMEN IN SET

Athena Factor 2.0: Accelerating Female Talent in Science,
Engineering & Technology
Sponsors: American Express, Boehringer Ingelheim USA,
BP, Genentech, McKesson Corporation, Merck Serono,
Schlumberger, Siemens AG (2014)

The Under-Leveraged Talent Pool: Women Technologists on
Wall Street
Sponsors: Bank of America, Credit Suisse, Goldman Sachs,
Intel, Merrill Lynch, NYSE Euronext (2008)

Stopping the Exodus of Women in Science
Harvard Business Review, June 2008

The Athena Factor: Reversing the Brain Drain in Science,
Engineering, and Technology
Sponsors: Alcoa, Cisco, Johnson & Johnson, Microsoft, Pfizer
(2008)

INDEX OF EXHIBITS

INDEX

TASK FORCE FOR TALENT INNOVATION

ABOUT THE AUTHOR

CAROLYN BUCK LUCE is senior managing director at Hewlett Consulting Partners and executive in residence at the Center for Talent Innovation, which she helped cofound with economist Sylvia Ann Hewlett. Formerly global pharmaceutical sector leader at Ernst & Young LLP, Buck Luce began her career as a diplomat and international investment banker. An adjunct professor at Columbia's Graduate School of International and Public Affairs and the coauthor of several *Harvard Business Review* articles, she is a recognized thought leader and dynamic speaker on the future of healthcare and women's leadership. In 2012, Buck Luce was named Woman of the Year by the Healthcare Businesswomen's Association. She graduated Phi Beta Kappa as well as magna cum laude from Georgetown University and received her MBA from Columbia University.